The answer to PCOS

By Norah Elizabeth Cozens

For all PCOS sufferers around the world.

My sincere wish is that you will use this book to its fullest. It has already helped thousands of PCOS sufferers and it can help you too.

Just follow the guidance to begin your road to recovery from the nightmare that is, PCOS.

You can do this for your hols April 24 Best Wishes Noral

© 2018 Norah Elizabeth Cozens
Cover design © 2018 Carrie Leaver

ISBN 978-1-5272-2582-4

All rights reserved. No part of this book may be reproduced, stored in a retrieval system or transmitted in any manner (including photocopying) without the express written permission of the author except for use in accordance with the provisions of the Copyright, Designs and Patents Act 1988.

Warning: The doing of an unauthorised act in relation to a copyright work may result in both a civil claim for damages and criminal prosecution.

Norah Elizabeth Cozens has asserted her moral rights in accordance with ss77-80 of the Copyright, Designs and Patents Act 1988.

Dedications

To Sasha and Andy McDonnell and the PCOS community who helped me devise this plan. Thank you for your enthusiasm and commitment to making a very traumatic journey for all of us, possible.

And to all PCOS sufferers everywhere who struggle every day with this devastating condition and need help to control their symptoms.

To my son, Damian, for his regular reminders to me of the need to get this book 'out there'.

Last but not least, to my late husband Francis who first had the idea for me to write a book on PCOS. It wasn't until 2010 when we were on a month's holiday in India, that I finally found time to sit down and write the first draft of this book. Francis' love, support and encouragement were, as always, unfailing.

Other books by Norah

Healthy Slimming Made Simple. First printed in 1980. Reprinted in 1984.
The 13 Minute Diet. First printed in 1989. Reprinted in 1992.

DISCLAIMER

The diet and lifestyle advice given in this book is not intended to replace the services of your doctor or any other health professional.

Following the advice and recommendations in this book is not a guarantee of increased fertility or pregacy.

You should always seek your doctor or other appropriately qualified health professional's advice before undertaking the diet or lifestyle recommendations in this book as your own physical condition and any medical diagnosis relating to your current or future health may require specific medications, precautions and/or other interventions.

For example, special precautions may be required if you are on medication for PCOS or under treatment for diabetes, infertility, thyroid disorder or any other medical or mental health condition, including (but not exclusively) depression, anxiety and eating disorders.

Any application of the suggestions, diets and procedures in this book is at your own discretion.

By following the advice in this book, it is understood that you accept this disclaimer.

Contents

About this book 8
Destiny leads me to PCOS 10
In the media spotlight 12
What's different about my plan? 14
Frequently asked questions on PCOS, weight loss and the diet 15

Chapter

1 Binge recovery & prevention 18
   - Binge busting 19
   - The binge barrier 20
   - Is this you? 21
   - Binge triggers and challenges 22
   - Bingeing — a very personal experience 27
   - Binge Recovery Guide 29
2 Finding out about PCOS 35
3 Fertility 41
4 Our miracle babies 46
5 Medical info 58
   PCOS symptoms and PCO 62
   Diagnosis, prevention and treatment 65
6 Before you start 69
   - Frequently asked questions about my plan 71
   - Guide to a 'good day' 76
   - More tips to improve weight loss 77
   - Your Sample Daily Food Tracker 78
   - What to do if you are constipated 79
   - Healthy habits to adopt 80

Contents (continued)

7	The diet — an introduction	84
	- The diet essentials	85
	- Your shopping list	86
	- Choose organic	87
	- Essential: Your Nibbles™ and Burns™	91
	- Frequently asked questions on Nibbles™ and Burns™	94
8	The 'new you' begins	95
	- The complete PCOS diet for immediate weight loss	96
	- What and how much to eat (includes meal plans)	98
9	Getting active	108
10	More life changing success stories	115
	- Sasha's story	117
	- Andy's story	120
	- Cheryl's story	124
	- Melissa's story	129
	- Emma's story	133
	- More success stories	135
11	The Maintenance Diet	139
12	Easy Soups & Sweets	147
	Guide to Eating Out	155
	Acknowledgements	160
	Image credits	161

About this book

This book is the culmination of my three years of trialling endless diets and lifestyle interventions to find out how to help PCOS (Polycystic Ovary Syndrome) sufferers who typically find it virtually impossible to lose weight and keep it off. It is without doubt, the pinnacle of my lifetime's work of over 40 years, successfully helping thousands of general slimmers lose weight and **keep it off!**

Amazingly, 97 out of 100 PCOS volunteers who painstakingly helped me develop my Healthy Eating and Lifestyle Plan for PCOS, reduced their PCOS symptoms enough to get pregnant. That's quite a result! Many had struggled for years with repeated miscarriages and in some cases, multiple IVFs; sadly, everything they'd tried had failed. (See 'Our miracle babies' on page 46 for pictures of just a few of the little ones I am so proud to have helped on their journey to planet Earth.)

Once you've been following my plan for a few weeks and lost weight you can find your hormones start to level out. So if you are struggling to get pregnant, this in itself can help you become more fertile. You should also check out the tips in my chapter on fertility — it's helped others; so why not you?

I've also included a much needed chapter on the sensitive subject of 'bingeing' to help tackle what is possibly the biggest barrier to weight loss. We've all been there; no matter how 'good' you've been all week; the 'binge monster' is always lurking in the background ready to whisper in your ear — 'go on eat it…one little cake won't hurt' — but we all know that one cake invariably leads to another and another and so on…threatening to destroy all the hard work you've put in to sticking to your diet. But fear not — help is at hand. I've included a copy of my tried and tested, Binge Recovery Guide. It will show you exactly how to rescue yourself from a binge and what you need to do to get bingeing under control, once and for all.

On my plan, there's no calorie counting or obsession with weighing and measuring everything — just a very brief list of foods that need to be restricted along with lists of the foods you should eat for maximum success. You'll also find lots of hints and tips to help you succeed along with a useful shopping list of all the basics you need to get started.

Meal plans for breakfast, lunch and evening meal are also included along with all you need to know about my Nibbles™ (vegetables) and Burns™ (proteins) — tiny pieces of food to be eaten every 15 minutes. They are ESSENTIAL to your success and will get you eating little and often to boost your metabolism and help you start losing weight, immediately.

For those of you who find moving around difficult; possibly because of weight or other health issues; you'll find the very easy, 5-minute daily exercises in the book very doable. They've been devised by a personal trainer so that almost anyone can do them. They can help boost your metabolism, improve your weight loss and tone your muscles. With caution and control, it is possible to use these exercises to take little 'steps' towards a physically fitter future.

And, if you find yourself thinking...'oh no, just another diet that won't work for me' ...then it's maybe time to think again. Thanks to some personal contributions from PCOS sufferers who've followed my plan, we get to share in some incredible, heartwarming success stories. Hats off to the contributors who've generously bared their souls so that PCOS 'cysters' everywhere can find the inspiration they need to follow my plan and begin their road to recovery from PCOS.

Please note: if you are one of those PCOS sufferers who does not have a weight problem but has other symptoms; you should read Natalie's story on page 52. PCOS has had a devastating impact on her life. She suffered traumas trying to get a diagnosis because she was slim, yet she has PCOS. After following my plan her symptoms reduced and she was able to eventually bring her precious children into the world. (For information on the symptoms of PCOS see the chapter on medical information on page 58.)

I've also included 'Andy's Story'; a lone voice in the book sharing what it's like to be the husband or partner of someone suffering with PCOS. Andy and his wife Sasha longed for a baby for many years until their dream came true. They've come through some of the most excessive, physical, mental and emotional trials of PCOS — a truly inspirational couple. (See their stories starting on page 117.)

Perhaps the most important thing, once you've lost the weight — is keeping it off! We all know that it's all too easy to find yourself back at 'square one' — very quickly. That's why I've included my Maintenance Diet. It will help to keep you on track by providing you with everything you need to say 'goodbye' to yo-yo dieting — forever!

And just as a little 'extra', you'll find a brief selection of my slimmers' favourite, super easy to prepare soups and sweets recipes, using everyday ingredients. I strongly recommend eating soup before main meals as a good way to pack a nutrient punch and feel fuller sooner. You'll also find the sweets recipes a great help for keeping on track when you're craving something sweet.

Finally, there's a 'Guide to Eating Out' so you know exactly what to eat when dining out, to stay on track.

Right now, there are millions of women with PCOS going through a living hell. This book has the answer. It shows how, in a matter of weeks, the symptoms of PCOS can be reduced so that sufferers can start to live healthier lives and avoid **the nightmare that is PCOS.**

Like thousands of slimmers before you, not just those with PCOS, I wish you every success with my plan and if you do get to hear the pitter patter of tiny feet as a result of following it — I'd love to know. I would also love to know if, after following my plan your PCOS symptoms reduce and your health improves. And, last but not least, how much weight you managed to lose. Just send an email to:
theanswertopcos@gmail.com so I can celebrate your success too.

Love, Norah

x

Destiny leads me to PCOS

My interest in health and fitness began over 40 years ago and grew from my own personal desire to maintain a healthy weight and learn as much as I could about keeping healthy.

To understand my own health, I studied nutrition and exercise and went on to develop my highly successful Healthy Eating and Lifestyle Plans which have helped thousands of slimmers in the UK and abroad lose weight and keep it off – no more yo-yo dieting!

In 1976 I launched 'Vitaline', my weight management company offering 1-2-1 nutritional guidance and support for slimmers. I sold that company in 2008 but have continued to support and advise slimmers ever since.

In 2001 I met Sasha McDonnell; a life-changing encounter that would lead me to develop my Healthy Eating and Lifestyle Plan for PCOS and eventually to write this book.

When I met Sasha she was struggling with her weight due to PCOS. She was also desperate for a baby but PCOS was causing her to have fertility issues.

By the time our paths crossed Sasha had all but given up hope of achieving her dream of motherhood. Her medical consultant told her to come back when she'd lost weight. But that was easier said than done. She'd struggled for years and had tried almost every diet known to man (and woman) but they simply did not work. She was at her wits' end and had no one professional to turn to; only her husband, family and friends.

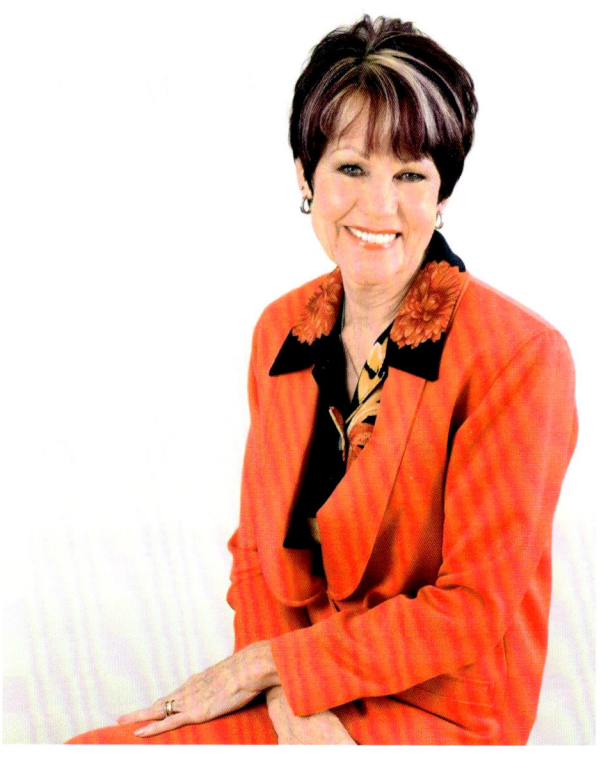

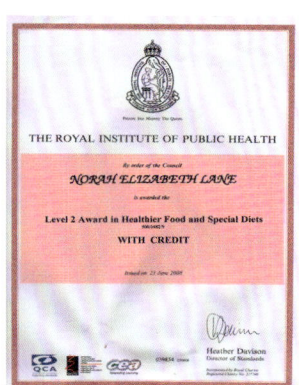

Norah's certificate in Healthier Food and Special Diets

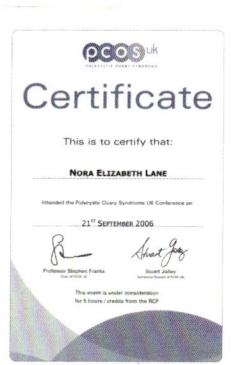

Norah's certificate of attendance: PCOS UK Conference

I was so moved by Sasha's story (see page 117) that I vowed silently to try and help her. It was quite an intimidating challenge, but I was determined to give it 'my all'. I felt instinctively, that the answer to managing PCOS must have something to do with diet and lifestyle choices – I just needed to find out what was happening to Sasha's body to see how they could make a difference.

First off, I approached specialists in female health to give me the benefit of their detailed knowledge and experience of PCOS. At the same time I launched trials into the impact of diet and lifestyle on PCOS sufferers. That took three years and involved 100 PCOS volunteers who underwent endless trials and testing. All of which led me to develop my Healthy Eating and Lifestyle Plan for PCOS.

It was quite a commitment from everyone. But I am delighted to say that in almost all cases, when followed diligently, my Healthy Eating and Lifestyle Plan for PCOS has been transformational. So much so that many of my PCOS clients' consultants, impressed by the vast improvements in both their patients' devastating symptoms and fertility, go on to recommend me to other of their PCOS patients.

Helping people from all walks of life lose weight and keep it off has been an incredible lifetime's journey. But being able to help PCOS women whose suffering and devastating symptoms are so often heartbreaking, see their symptoms reduce, enabling them to live a 'normal' life, has been extra specially rewarding.

Beyond that, the incredible feeling you get when a call comes through to say, 'Norah…I'm pregnant!' And then to share the anticipation of new life and the joy for a new mum and dad when their little miracle baby arrives: being a mum myself, I know that helping women achieve their dream of motherhood is something so very special.

This book is my third book on diets. The first is 'Healthy Slimming Made Simple', followed by the '13 Minute Diet'. I've also appeared many times on national TV and radio, presented lectures to hospitals on nutrition and PCOS and helped raise over £140,000 for worthy charitable causes.

But my work to help women suffering with PCOS has been the pinnacle. Time and time again, I hear from PCOS sufferers in despair telling me how they've got nowhere and no one to turn to for help; many suffering unbearably for years.

If you are suffering from PCOS, I encourage you to follow my Healthy Eating and Lifestyle Plan for PCOS — you will be so glad you did.

Love, Norah

x

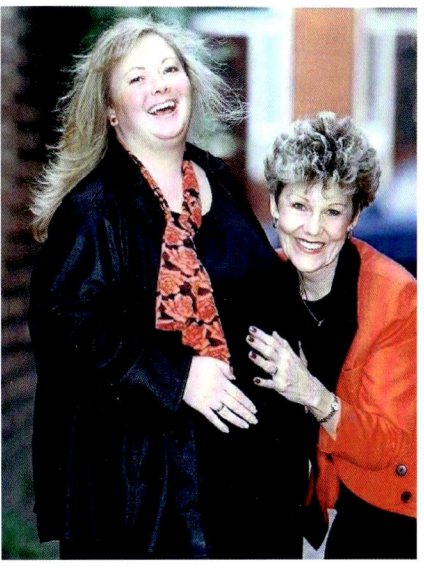

After years of trying — Libby McDonnell, Norah's first PCOS baby, is on the way — Mum-to-be Sasha and Norah are absolutely thrilled

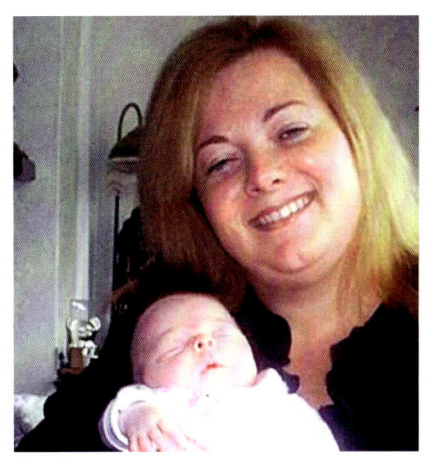

Sasha cuddling Libby: our first miracle

In the media spotlight

Over the years, I have made numerous radio and TV appearances to share the benefits of my Healthy Eating and Lifestyle Plan. But the way it all started came as a bit of a surprise. To tell you the story, I need to go back to July 2007.

My husband Francis and I were driving down to London for a much needed weekend break. We'd been driving for about an hour when my mobile phone rang. The voice on the other end said. 'Is that Norah? I work for the Daily Express and I want to talk to you about your diet.'

I wasn't expecting a call from the media so naturally, I thought it was a friend or family member messing about. Eventually the journalist persuaded me that he really was from the newspaper. He went on to explain that my diet had been selected for its success and was in the paper.

'..my diet had been selected for its success and was in the paper.'

I was thrilled! He went on to explain that I should also be aware that the story of my success had been published and that I would be front page news in today's paper with details of the diet spread across two inside pages (12th July 2007).

He apologised for not telling me in advance; as is the usual protocol at the paper but, somehow that job had fallen between the cracks on an extremely busy newsroom floor.

Next stop was the motorway services station where we picked up a few copies of the newspaper. It was a real thrill to see we'd made it into the national press; and without even trying!

All manner of newspapers, magazines, TV and radio stations soon followed; helping me to spread the word. Before all the publicity we were doing very well locally, but the wider exposure meant we were able to help people up and down the country and outside the UK.

Obesity is a common symptom of PCOS. It's also becoming more and more of a problem in the general population. In fact, there's never been a more obese period in human history; so much so that many countries are bracing themselves for an obesity epidemic. It's even predicted that future generations of parents will outlive their obese children, if we don't do something soon.

So, whilst this book is dedicated to helping PCOS sufferers, I can help general slimmers too with other Healthy Eating and Lifestyle Plans — for more information please send an email to **theanswertopcos@gmail.com**.

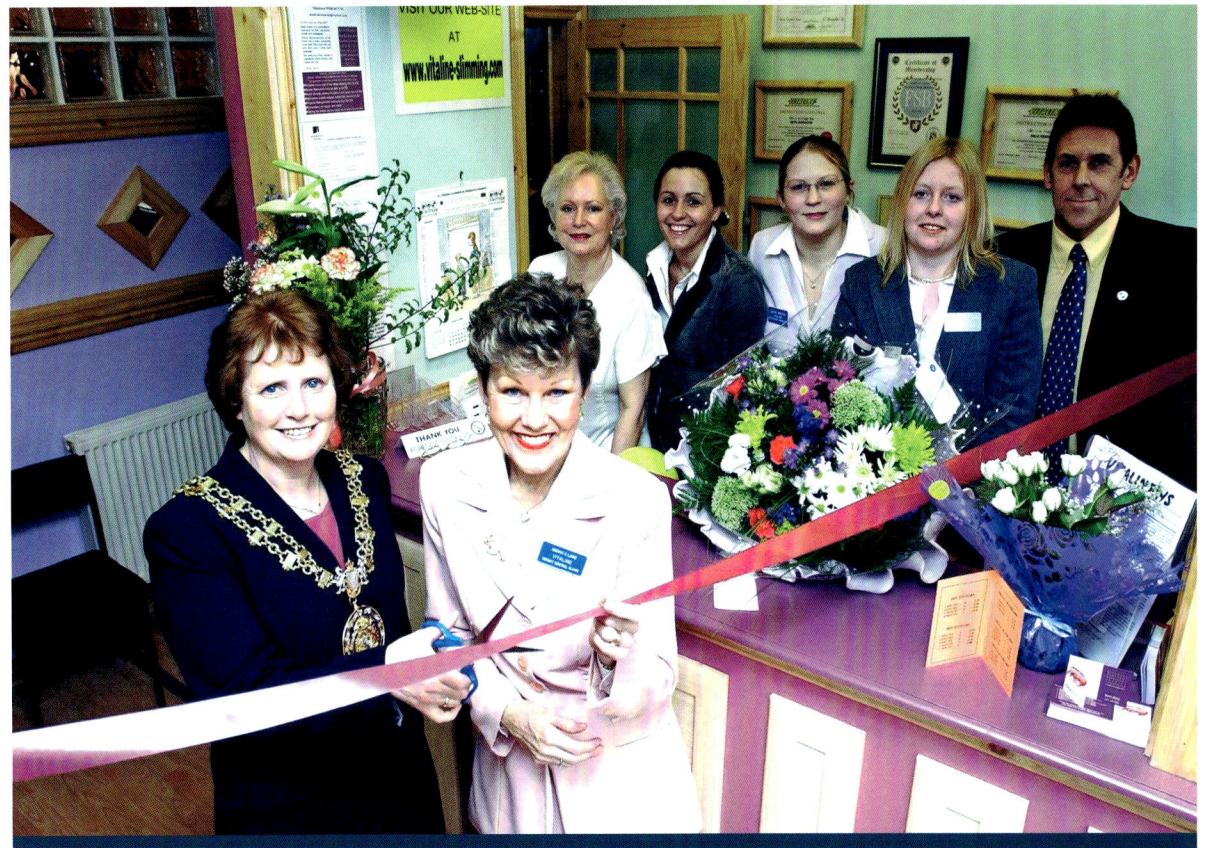

Posing for the local press: The ex-Mayoress of Tameside (Pauline Harrison) opening Norah's new Vitaline Clinic in Denton in the North of England

So far I have had over 1,000 babies born to mothers who followed my plan, many of whom struggled for years to get pregnant.

I would love to hear from you if after following my Healthy Eating and Lifestyle Plan for PCOS, you become pregnant. Judging by the outcome of my trials into the impact of diet and lifestyle on PCOS (see page 35), where 97 out of 100 of my volunteers became pregnant; the number of new babies born in the future could be phenomenal!

I'd also love to hear from you if you've found my plan has helped your unpleasant PCOS symptoms reduce and how successful your weight loss has been.

To let me know, please send an email to:
theanswertopcos@gmail.com

What's different about my plan?

PCOS sufferers have a unique set of challenges to health and to losing weight. These include hormone and chemical imbalances that can lead to cravings and regular binges. It is therefore essential that chemicals and food additives are eliminated from the diet wherever possible. That's why I recommend eating only real, fresh, organic food (if possible).

On this diet:

- **You must eat to lose weight**
- **You will be eating much more than usual**
- **You will never be hungry (unless you have an extraordinarily large appetite)**

Plastic containers used to heat food are also to be avoided along with processed foods to minimise the absorption of unnatural substances. Drinking from plastic bottles that may have been near heat or left lying in the sun (usually in cars) is also inadvisable.

The diet is laid out in meal format. All you do is select your choice of breakfast, lunch, evening meal and supper snack from your diet menu. This makes it easy to follow and can result in a good weight loss every week.

The plan:

- Is based on my original Healthy Eating and Lifestyle Plan which has evolved over more than 40 years and incorporates what I learned during my three years of trialling diet and lifestyle with over 100 PCOS volunteers

- Uses only fresh produce, including high quality animal protein, all freely available in shops and supermarkets

- Relies on organic foods wherever possible because they contain fewer pesticides and chemicals

- Uses my patented Nibbles™ and Burns™ system to boost metabolism every 15 minutes, ensuring that slimmers eat little and often — the key to the plan's success

- Includes my Binge Recovery Guide — an essential tool for all slimmers but especially PCOS slimmers because hormonal imbalances mean they can crave carbohydrates and starches

- Includes my Maintenance Diet to help keep the weight off once it has been lost

- Has helped women with PCOS improve their fertility — over 1,000 babies have been born to women often desperate to be mothers, many of whom struggled for years to have a baby

Because some of the medicines prescribed to PCOS sufferers can deplete B vitamins in the body, this diet is rich in organic animal protein which is an excellent source of these vitamins.

Frequently asked questions on PCOS, weight loss and the diet

What is PCOS?

PCOS is a medical condition linked to hormonal imbalance and insulin resistance. It affects four in every twenty women.

How do I know I have PCOS?

If you have symptoms like excessive weight gain, ovulation or fertility problems, period problems, facial or bodily hair, mood swings, acne, tiredness, thinning hair, cravings for food, skin tags, depression, irritability, a tendency to faint or emotional problems; you could have PCOS.

Your doctor should arrange an ultrasound scan and a blood test to determine if you have PCOS. Remember you don't need to have all the symptoms, you may have only two or three and still have PCOS.

Is there a cure for PCOS?

No. But the good news is that PCOS sufferers can manage their symptoms and lead perfectly healthy lives if they keep their weight under control, take regular exercise and make appropriate lifestyle changes.

Will I always have a weight problem because of PCOS?

You can lose weight; many PCOS sufferers struggle to lose weight because one of the symptoms of PCOS is a slow metabolism.

My Healthy Eating and Lifestyle Plan for PCOS, designed to speed up your metabolism, has been helping PCOS sufferers for over 17 years. If you follow my recommendations, you can lose weight consistently until you reach your desired weight.

Will I be able to have children with PCOS?

Some PCOS sufferers have fertility problems. Your medical consultant will explain the many options available. The success rate for conception is increasing all the time.

Over 1,000 babies have been born to my PCOS slimmers to date. All had been struggling to get pregnant before following my Healthy Eating and Lifestyle Plan for PCOS. By losing weight, reducing their symptoms, eating nutritious food and boosting their metabolism, they were able to give themselves an excellent chance of getting pregnant, naturally.

Why do I find it difficult to lose weight with PCOS?

PCOS is a chemical or hormone imbalance, linked to insulin resistance. This can make losing weight very difficult for many sufferers. Many PCOS sufferers are also 'carbohydrate sensitive'. They can crave carbohydrates with many sufferers being unable to stop eating foods like sugars, and certain starchy carbohydrates. PCOS sufferers also typically have a sluggish metabolism.

Because of an insulin resistance problem, your diet needs to be low sugar, low fat, low carbohydrate with good quality animal protein, and plenty of fruit and vegetables. Animal protein is a good source of essential vitamins. You may especially need foods containing B vitamins because some PCOS medications can deplete B vitamins in the body. These vitamins need replacing for good health.

Why do I need organic food?

When you suffer with PCOS it is important that you keep your food and drinks chemical free. Organic food is better because it is additive free and will not affect the balance of chemicals in your body.

What type of diet is it?

It's much more than just a diet — it's a special Healthy Eating and Lifestyle Plan for PCOS sufferers. It's not restrictive and is designed to increase your metabolism and cater to your preferred eating habits and lifestyle.

You will eat little and often so you will not be hungry on this diet. It will contain all the vitamins and minerals you need to lose weight and can help you reduce your PCOS symptoms. Once you have reached your desired weight, you can use the Maintenance Diet (see page 139) to keep the weight off permanently.

What kind of food is on the diet?

Everyday foods, but preferably organic. Your diet will contain a choice of breakfasts, lunches, evening meals and snacks for when you feel hungry.

Because you suffer from PCOS the diet will be low fat, low sugar, low carbohydrate with plenty of good quality animal protein, fruit and vegetables. The protein food will provide the vitamins that are essential to your health.

The diet is very easy to follow. I provide a list of all the foods you need to help speed up your metabolism and help you lose weight faster. Once you are losing weight successfully, you can introduce a daily treat if you like!

Can I drink alcohol, eat takeaways and dine in restaurants on the diet?

Yes. You can have a glass of red wine occasionally. Red wine contains bioflavanoids which are good for your heart. You can also eat in restaurants and have takeaways providing you choose wisely, eat sensibly and steer clear of foods with additives or chemicals. See page 155 for more tips on eating out.

How much weight can I lose on the diet?

If you have more than 19 kg/42 lbs to lose, you can expect to lose at least 2.5 kg/5 lbs in your first week, then a regular 1 kg/2 lbs a week after that. Doctors recommend a slow weight loss so that excess fat is lost rather than muscle.

How can you help me stop 'cheating' on the plan?

I've devised a Binge Recovery Guide, based on the real-life experiences of the PCOS volunteers who were part of my diet and lifestyle trials into PCOS (see pages 29 and 35). The Guide will help you avoid cheating.

Will my PCOS symptoms reduce if I lose weight?

Yes. My PCOS clients have reported significant reductions in their symptoms after losing weight. Some clients have been told by their medical consultant or medical practitioners that their weight loss has resulted in their cysts shrinking.

The benefits of losing weight can be transformational. For example, your hair can become thicker; if you suffer with acne, your skin can improve; your mood swings can become less frequent; your periods can return and be less painful; your confidence can improve and your chances of getting pregnant can increase; if that is your aim.

Do I need to exercise whilst dieting?

Exercising within your own capabilities is good for you but never needs to be strenuous. See my simple exercises, devised by a personal trainer on page 108. They can be performed in the comfort and privacy of your own home, with very little effort. Naturally, it helps if you can keep active doing everyday things like walking and gardening or going swimming. The more you move the more calories you will burn off.

If I crave sweet foods, do I need to give them up?

No. There is a selection of sweets recipes (see page 153) for the times when you want something sweet but don't want to go off the rails.

Do I have to weigh and measure all my foods?

I appreciate that there isn't always time to weigh foods. That's one of the reasons my diet is laid out in meal format. All you do is select your choice of breakfast, lunch, evening meal and supper snack from your diet menu. This makes it easy to follow and manage and will result in a good weight loss every week.

Chapter One
Bingeing

Recovery & prevention

Binge busting

The importance of getting to grips with bingeing cannot be emphasised enough.

Bingeing is the most destructive force when you are trying to lose weight and one that is a real challenge for any slimmer, particularly PCOS slimmers.

This is therefore, probably, the most important chapter in this book because without a way of busting out of bingeing; you will struggle to succeed.

Please be sure to read everything in here; and follow it up by using my Binge Recovery Guide every day. It will help you break bad habits around bingeing and form much better, healthier ones.

Good luck with your binge recovery! You can do it!

Love Norah

x

In this chapter

The binge barrier

Is this you?

Binge triggers and challenges

Bingeing — a very personal experience

The binge barrier

If you find yourself thinking... 'not another book on PCOS; I've read loads and I still can't get any help – and I can't stop bingeing so it's useless trying to diet...' then please wait until you hear me out.

We all know that binge eating is one of the most difficult subjects to talk about. People often feel disgusted and ashamed of themselves after a binge. But at the same time, it's sort of an open secret that no-one feels comfortable admitting to doing it.

It's all linked to how people feel about themselves and if left to run riot, bingeing will only cause harm to a person both psychologically and physically.

For PCOS slimmers, the battle can be that much harder because of their daily struggle with mood swings and depression, caused by hormonal imbalances.

And, it's precisely because bingeing is so destructive and such a big barrier to successful weight loss that we should 'talk' about it from the start.

It's such a serious problem that you may even find that in addition to foods like pies, bread, pasta and rice, you find yourself bingeing on foods you don't normally like; just because they are there!

If this is familiar to you then please don't despair...you are not alone. Slimmers everywhere, not just PCOS slimmers, often have a daily battle with binge eating. But, if you suffer with PCOS the desire to binge could be even more challenging. Mood swings and depression are generally behind the impulse to binge; triggered usually by an emotional 'event'.

> 'Because of my devastating PCOS symptoms and obesity, I felt ugly. My sex life with my partner had come to an end as I was embarrassed to be seen undressed.
>
> 'My partner and I were leading separate lives and were about to split up, when a friend told me about this diet plan. She was also a PCOS sufferer. I decided to give it a go as I had tried everything else and had nothing to lose. My life was in a mess.
>
> 'Within three months, I lost three stone, became much more confident and happier as the symptoms started to diminish. I now enjoy life to the full, with my partner.
>
> 'The Binge Recovery Guide was an essential part of my success.
>
> 'Thank you Norah for this amazing healthy eating plan.'
>
> **Mary, London**

Is this you?

Let's take a closer look...

Does this sound like you? You've had a bad day. Your PCOS symptoms are getting you down and you just don't know how you are ever going to cope with all the problems they are causing you. Worse still, you've starved yourself for a week and not lost an ounce. Feeling low you drive to the nearest petrol station to buy a multipack of chocolate bars; you take them home and eat the lot in one go.

You've just finished the last of them... two minutes later you find yourself reaching for your car keys to go and get some more. There's no way you're going back to the same petrol station, that would be mortifying. So instead you drive over to a different petrol station. The next thing you know is you're sitting on your sofa surrounded by six more empty wrappers from the chocolate bars.

You gather them up and do a thorough check around to make sure you haven't left any wrappers anywhere for someone to find. You look for somewhere to hide them and decide to put them in your handbag for when you're passing a bin on the high street.

The following emotions are highly likely to trigger a binge

Do you feel: trapped, powerless, frustrated, disappointed, unfairly burdened, unattractive or unloved, heartbroken, hopeless, desperate, or in some extreme cases, suicidal?

With PCOS you can be on an unending emotional roller coaster with your feelings about life and about yourself changing from day to day. It could be that a friend tells you she's pregnant. She's already got one baby while you, after years of trying and endless negative pregnancy tests, still haven't been able to conceive.

These are the kinds of emotional events where my Binge Recovery Guide will really help you. Using the Guide will help you to stay in close touch with the way you are feeling; hour by hour. It gives doable, practical advice on how to avert a binge; encouraging you to monitor your progress each and every day until YOU are in complete control.

If bingeing is a problem for you; you are not alone (rest assured, I am the last person to judge; because like everyone else, I've been there too).

Many of my PCOS slimmers (and general slimmers too) have used my Binge Recovery Guide and found that with the focus and determination to use it fully, they've been able to stop bingeing.

Love, Norah x

Binge triggers and challenges

It is possible to put an end to bingeing...but you will have to commit to managing bingeing by working at preventing it EVERY DAY! **And because nothing is effective 100% of the time, you will need to focus hard to succeed.**

Take action by following my Binge Recovery Guide. Make sure you also use the Binge Recovery Diary to help you identify your triggers and monitor your progress and successes (see page 32). You should also review the Common Binge Triggers' table on page 33. Do you recognise some of these triggers? Knowing what your triggers are will help you avoid them.

Keep a record of your triggers and score them as suggested in the examples. Score how well you managed them and make other detailed notes as suggested in the examples. It will really help you conquer bingeing, especially if you rate your successes, (between 1-10) along the way. Doing well will be a strong incentive to keep going when the going gets tough. My Binge Recovery Guide has been tried, and tested by the 100 volunteers who trialled endless diets and lifestyle interventions over a three year period as well as thousands of PCOS sufferers since...and it works! Everything in my Binge Recovery Guide is there because my volunteers proved its value in helping them conquer bingeing. **Remember: With patience and commitment, you can achieve great things!**

The first thing to do to aid your binge recovery, make up an 'emergency box' of food which you keep in the fridge for when you are tempted. A good time to prepare your emergency food is soon after finishing a meal.

Here are some of the most common binge triggers and challenges and how to handle them.

I am having a really bad day. I feel really down and I'm in the kitchen looking for something to binge on — so I can feel better!

This is how to rescue yourself from a binge:

Step 1: Make a warm drink.

Step 2: Get out of the kitchen.

Step 3: Resolve not to eat anything for ten minutes.

Step 4: Go into the lounge and put on some soothing music.

Step 5: Sit down in a comfortable chair with your feet up.

Step 6: Drink it slowly, savour every mouthful of your drink.

Step 7: After you've finished, close your eyes and relax.

Within five minutes that awful 'panic feeling' will have gone and you will feel a real sense of satisfaction because now you can say:

'I've managed to control my first eating binge after years of bingeing and going completely out of control.'

After relaxing for ten minutes, if you feel hungry go back into the kitchen, take out your 'emergency box' and eat the prepared food, but take it back into the lounge – **never eat in the kitchen!**

I've been doing well recently…not bingeing…but I feel I could give in quite easily!

Give yourself a score based on how well you managed a binge. Award yourself out of 10.

Fill in your Binge Recovery Diary – that way – when you have a bad day, you can see how well you've coped and what you did to avoid bingeing. You'll also be able to 'see' how well you are doing…how few 'bad days' you are having – that in itself could motivate you **not** to binge.

Make sure you write in your Binge Recovery Diary 'when' you prepare your emergency food…ideally just after you've had a meal…and **never** when you are hungry. It is a good habit that will keep you conscious of doing all the things you need to do to avert a binge.

Assuming you've already prepared your 'emergency food', when you approach your usual cheating time – **recognise** you are going out of control. The 'panic' feeling will not disappear unless you control it.

> When you need to be reminded how far you've come or why what you are doing for yourself is so worthwhile, try and focus on the positive things in your life. You will be getting your life back on track by following my Healthy Eating and Lifestyle Plan for PCOS.

I just don't get why it's important to record all this information about my life!

Now the MOST important part!

Fill in your Binge Recovery Diary every day. It really is important for PCOS sufferers to stay in touch with their feelings and binge triggers. Because of hormonal imbalances you are likely to struggle every day with cravings and mood swings, if not depression or other phsychological issues such as anxiety. Don't forget to award yourself a score for how well you managed your binge. By referring back to it at a later date, you'll realise that you are actually cutting down on your binges.

This is how you will learn to stop using food as a substitute for other things, such as affection, love and boredom.

If you tend to binge because of pre-menstrual tension (this can happen even if your periods are absent), you will be able to prepare mentally and practically for this 'bad time' and take action to avoid bingeing.

I'm always busy. Running from here to there, trying to do everything...not just for me...everyone around me seems to need me. I can't cope with the demand it's exhausting...I never have any 'me' time.

Everyone is busy these days but beware...if you are continually 'doing for others', you will eventually feel like a martyr.

It could lead to feelings of resentment and drive you to eating a 'cheat'. It's far better to allow a little time to yourself every day, you will feel so much better for it.

I am so busy, I don't have time to eat!

Don't miss meals. As a PCOS sufferer, if you go too long without food, your blood sugar levels start to drop. This will make you feel very low and could result in a binge.

I often feel hungry between meals.

If you feel hungry between meals, have one of the snacks suggested in my Healthy Eating and Lifestyle Plan for PCOS (see page 96).

I am always forgetting my Burns™ or Nibbles™.

Set an alarm on your phone if you can and eat a Burn™ or a Nibble™ every 15 minutes to keep you away from the biscuit barrel. It's best to get them ready at the beginning of the day so they're there ready for you.

I can't help craving for things like pasta and bread with loads of butter and jam.

Try to avoid having any fattening foods in the house, just don't buy them...they will only tempt you. Butter is fine as you need some fat every day but only within your daily allowance. If you don't buy fattening foods everyone in the house will benefit healthwise.

It's hard not to eat what my husband eats for his dinner. Buttery mash, fried pork chops and loads of onions and gravy — and don't even mention the microwave lasagnes he loves.

Encourage healthy-eating for your partner/husband...it's the best way you can avoid being tempted. They will benefit too with healthier choices.

> Controlling your cravings will have enormous psychological benefits. Remember the numerous times you've woken up in the morning thinking about food and gone to bed at night thinking about food? Not any longer. Following my Binge Recovery Guide will help you put food into perspective. You'll see that controlling your obsession with carbohydrates and sugars will transform your life...you'll feel good about yourself and 'know' you have the power to change it for good.

Because I am trying to lose weight I try and limit myself and keep my food simple to the point of it being quite boring.

Most PCOS sufferers get fed up because they are bored with dull and uninteresting food. You need to make sure you are varying your food but rest assured you will enjoy your food on my Healthy Eating and Lifestyle Plan for PCOS. By varying it too, you will give your metabolism a boost. Why not try the tasty soups and sweets recipes on page 147.

I find doing exercise boring. But I know it's good for me.

Exercise is known as a mood booster because it releases endorphins or happy hormones. Try and find an exercise you enjoy or at least go for walks – it will be good for your all round health.

I keep buying treats whenever I pop to the shops for some groceries...I know I shouldn't but I can't help it when they always put chocolates near the tills.

Plan your food ahead by deciding what you are going to eat so you can do all your shopping at one time. Take along a list of your allowed foods and only buy what's on that. When you have food in the house that you *can* eat, you will be far less tempted to cheat. Take some fruit with you to eat when you go shopping and enjoy healthy fruit instead. You will be glad you did.

I find it especially difficult not to binge when I'm feeling low. I can easily eat my way through two packets of chocolate biscuits – then I feel disgusted with myself.

Make a list of jobs to do during the times you have noted you are most likely to binge. When you feel a binge coming on do a job from your list. Tick it off when done. *You* will have changed a destructive 'binge time' into a constructive and productive 'event'.

The sense of satisfaction it will give you will be tremendous and give you strength for another day. Weeks later, when you read your Binge Recovery Diary you will realise just how much time you wasted on bingeing and how much more productive and in control you are now.

As one PCOS sufferer told us:

'The list of jobs I completed, really made me feel good.'

Ideas that can help

Here are just 10 suggestions — pick any one to keep you away from the biscuit barrel or...make up your own 'go to' list for when you feel tempted:

1. Housework
2. Buy some more houseplants
3. Try your hand at arts & crafts
4. Organise your wardrobe
5. Have a clearout and donate to your local charity shop
6. Frame some photos you've been planning for ages
7. Tidy your bookshelves
8. Try 'upcycling' an old chair
9. Refresh the paint in a room of your house or flat
10. Arrange a coffee morning with friends

'Norah knows everything about PCOS. She helped me to control my cravings for carbohydrates with her binge recovery guide.'
Ann, Cheshire

Bingeing – a very personal experience

'It's like two people inside you. One is saying 'NO you must resist', whilst the other is saying, 'go on, that little piece of cake or slice of bread won't matter', and then it happens. You go on a binge. You eat everything in sight, sometimes even food that you don't really like. You are like something out of control. After the binge, you regret what you have done, feel disgusted with yourself, have a cry, get depressed and off you go again.'

Jane, PCOS slimmer

Start your binge free life!

To help you live a binge free life, I have devised the following Guide so you can manage cravings and ditch binge eating **forever**!

Tried and tested by my PCOS clients, my Binge Recovery Guide will help get you back on your Healthy Eating and Lifestyle Plan for PCOS. You'll be left with a tremendous feeling of satisfaction knowing you have conquered those terrible eating binges **once and for all!**

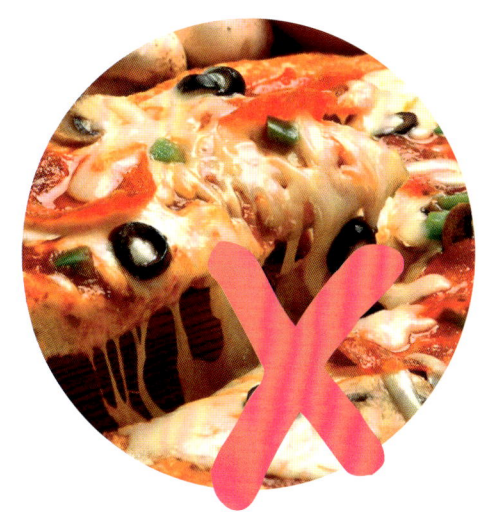

Health benefit: Statistics prove that you are likely to live a good deal longer, be less susceptible to heart disease and high blood pressure, if you eat healthily and your weight is normal. It's never too late to take action... but sooner is better than later.

Get a hobby and ...make a list of all the things you need/like to do

Sometimes temptation can be everywhere; especially if you are craving or upset about something. When this happens, distract yourself and do something you enjoy or something that gets you out of the house and away from the kitchen!

Make a list of all the things you need to do such as ironing or clearing out cupboards (see previous page for some suggestions). When you've done a job note it, 'with pride' in your Binge Recovery Diary. **You've just turned a destructive potential binge into a constructive, positive 'event' — well done!**

You'll feel **empowered** and **in control** — not battling the binge monster!

All of this can help in a moment of weakness to keep you occupied and take your mind off all negative thoughts that could lead to a binge — it is a vital part of your success so please do give it your all.

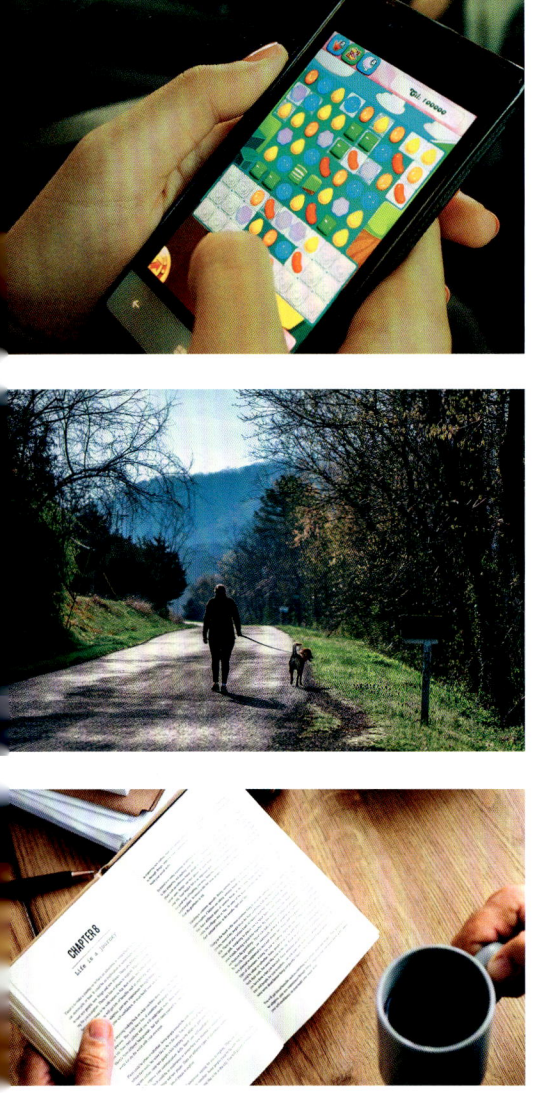
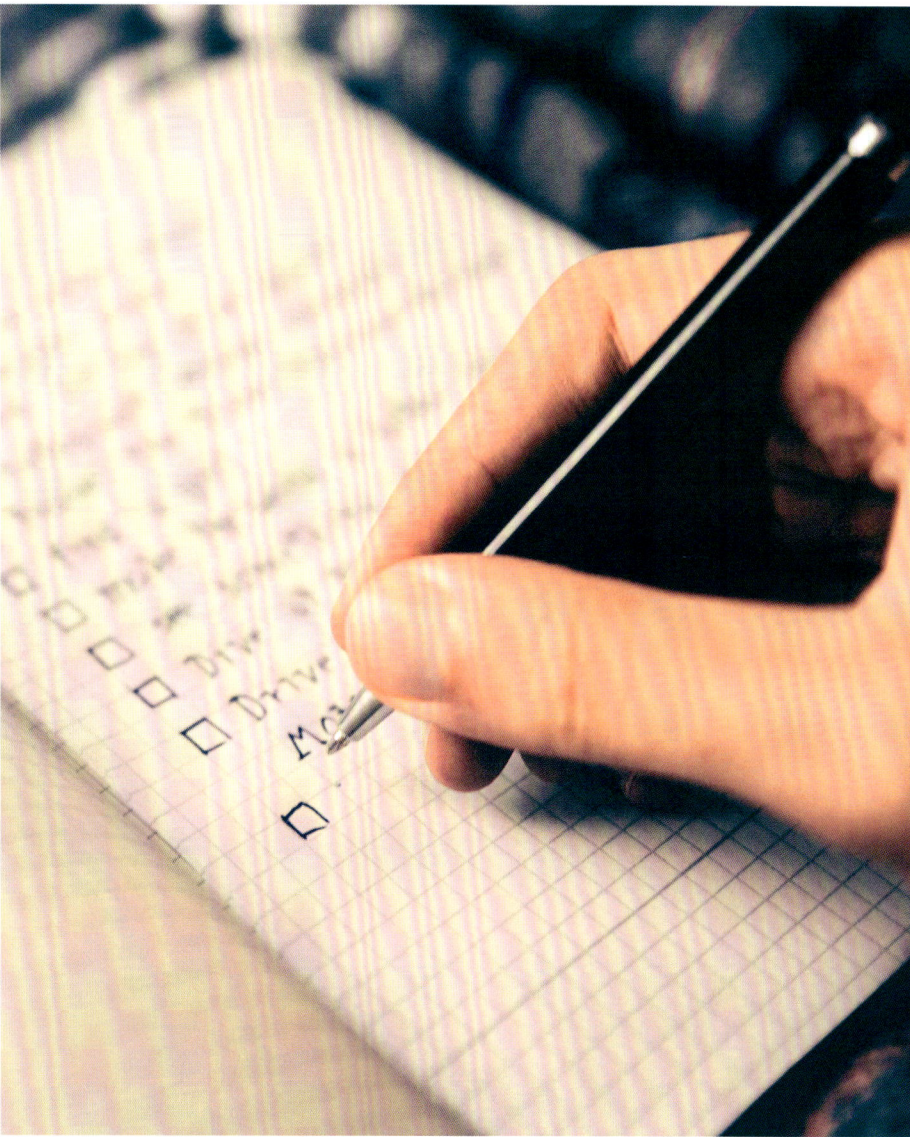

Binge Recovery Guide

Your master key

This Binge Recovery Guide is the key to mastering bingeing. It has been tried and tested and developed to give you all the tools you need to really understand your bingeing habit. That is an important step because bingeing is a very personal experience and must start with you really understanding what happens in your life that triggers a binge.

With the daily practise of using the Guide you will find that you really can stop bingeing...which means if you are determined enough...that can mean you can stop FOREVER!

There isn't a slimmer on the planet who hasn't at some stage during a diet, gone 'wolf' on a barrel of biscuits — I know, I've done it too!

So, don't hesitate...I want you to use this Guide every day until you have mastered bingeing. That way your chances of success will multiply and soon you will be able to say; **'I did it! — the binge monster no longer has any power over me.**'

In this chapter

Taking control

Sample binge recovery diary

Be alert — what are your binge triggers?

Celebrate your success and give yourself an incentive

Taking control

I think we all agree that food should be a pleasure; not something destructive. But for PCOS sufferers binge eating can be a common, damaging experience.

During my three year diet and lifestyle trials into their impact on PCOS (see page 35) I discovered that eating foods containing chemicals, additives or colourings (most foods contain at least one of these) aggravates hormone imbalances; one of the major problems associated with PCOS. This is the reason PCOS sufferers tend to crave foods like sugars and starches. Not only is bingeing bad for you, it can seriously impact your healthy eating regime, throwing you right off course — all the more reason to take control.

This Binge Recovery Guide will help you take control of your cravings and emotional triggers. As bingeing is often a big challenge for PCOS sufferers; something they may battle with every day; it is really important that you make a habit of staying in touch with your feelings. Spend time reviewing how well you are doing; especially when you feel you are about to start craving something. If you can stay in touch with your feelings and your cravings, you will soon find you are in control and can conquer bingeing forever.

Keys to your success

1. Type up your Binge Recovery Diary and make sure you fill it in every day (see the example on page 32). This is critically important. It will help you keep in touch with the way you are feeling. This is so important for those who suffer mood swings/and or depression because they can more often than not, lead to bingeing.

2. Find things you like to do that will keep you mentally and physically occupied. If you don't already have one, get a hobby – it's a great way to distract yourself when you feel a binge coming on.

3. Always keep some healthy snacks ready prepared in the fridge. This is your **emergency food** and is best prepared when you're not hungry, say after dinner; **never when hungry!**

4. When you binge, analyse the times and reasons. That way you can plan ahead to avoid a binge. Be sure to write these details down in your Binge Recovery Diary.

5. Weigh yourself at the same time of the day, once a week only, on accurate scales that sit flat on the floor.

Sample Binge Recovery Diary (type up and fill in every time you have had a binge or been tempted!)

Date 29 April 2018	Sample answers
Time binge began (there's always a pattern, e.g. evenings/weekends)	9.30pm
What did I binge on?	Bought a packet of chocolate biscuits on my way home from work
How much did I eat?	Ate them all
What triggered my binge?	My period is taking forever to arrive My friend just told me she's pregnant and we've been trying for years! Not been sticking to the diet so no weight lost for a while I had a row with my mother
What could I have done to avoid bingeing?	I could have visited my granddad. Living alone, he gets very lonely. We always have a cuppa and he tells me things about my grandma and about my mum growing up — should have focused on his needs not mine
What stopped me bingeing?	Someone called at the house I had a phone call from my friend
How did I feel when my binge was over?	More depressed than ever :(
How is the Binge Recovery Guide helping me?	I feel much better about things Not disgusted with myself I'm on my way to stopping bingeing
When did I prepare my emergency food?	After dinner
How's my attitude to bingeing changing?	I now know what triggers a binge so I try and pre-empt them Now I've always got my emergency food in the fridge
Score how well you are conquering bingeing using the guide below*.	7
Which job did I do to avert a binge? (See suggestions on previous page.)	Cleaned the bathroom tiles

*Binge Scoring Guide

1 = I went overboard — ate five bars of chocolate
2 = Very conscious that I need to get control
3 = Only half a binge
4 = Beginning to 'own' my binges
5 = Didn't binge as much as I used to

6 = I am definitely getting stronger
7 = Getting better at distracting myself
8 = Nearly in control
9 = Amazingly well — but not quite there
10 = Stopped myself bingeing

Be alert — what are your binge triggers?

Take some time to think about what triggers you to binge. Try to think of ways of minimising their impact so you don't get thrown off course.

Common Binge Triggers	What to do
You are feeling depressed	Try and focus on someone else — maybe an elderly relative who is lonely and could do with a catch up over a cup of tea or simply a hand with tasks at home. Even a telephone call to them will help
You discover a friend is pregnant and although you try and be happy for her, deep inside your longing for your own child is overwhelming	Try and focus on the positive things in your life and how you are getting your life back. My diet is designed to boost your metabolism and nourish your body while you are losing weight. The good news is it can help to level out your hormones and give you a chance of getting pregnant
My period is taking forever to arrive and I've had pre-menstrual tension for ages	Being well organised so that you can get through your chores and manage your day well will give you time to dedicate to you and managing your feelings. Treat yourself to a spa session or a manicure
I am feeling nervous/anxious	Spend some time resting. Clear your mind and try and focus on listening to your breath. Breathing in for three counts; hold for three counts and breathe out for three counts. Repeat a couple of times — this will help to relax you
I am worried about something	Try not to worry — try and find a distraction to take your mind off whatever is worrying you. Don't allow worrying to lead to a binge, sabotaging all your efforts to eat healthy food
I had a row with my husband/mother/sister	Try to avoid rows and heightened emotion. If things are getting heated it's best to keep calm and remember you are on a healthy eating mission and nothing or no one is going to jeopardise your success — if you can, take yourself out of the situation

Celebrate your success and give yourself an incentive!

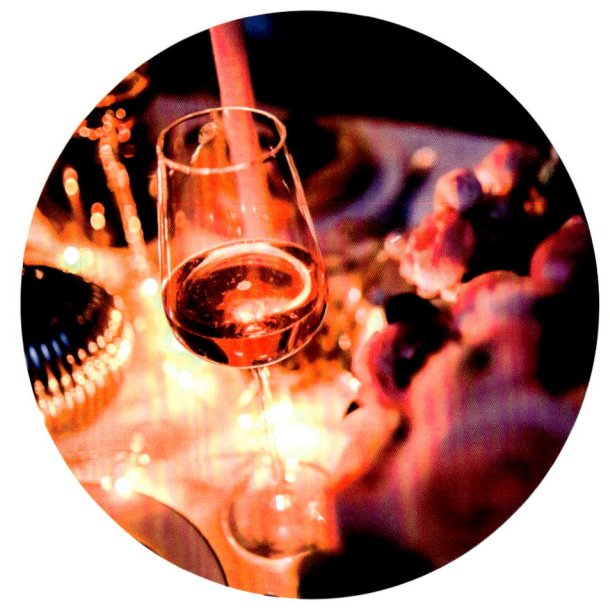

When you've done well over time and avoided bingeing...give yourself a special treat. Do something for you! It is important psychologically to recognise your achievements.

Maybe get a manicure or plan a really healthy meal for you and your partner or a friend...incentives are a great way to keep you on track (see my Guide to Eating Out on page 155).

'You've taught me more about my PCOS condition in the last 45 minutes than I've learned in the last thirty odd years from any doctor. Now I know I've found someone I can trust and rely on to help me. Thank you Norah!'

Jenny, Manchester

Chapter Two
Finding out about PCOS

Learning how to help

When I made a silent vow to help PCOS sufferer Sasha McDonnell (see page 10), I began a heartfelt mission to find the link between diet and lifestyle, and PCOS. Little did I know then that it would take me three years to learn which diet and lifestyle interventions would help PCOS sufferers lose weight and/or reduce their symptoms.

With endless trials to set up and review, it was a real rollercoaster ride at times, but worth all the ups and downs because the plan has helped thousands of sufferers so successfully.

Although it only really scratches the surface of the work I did, this chapter gives a brief overview of what was involved in finding my answer to PCOS.

The success of my three years of trialling diet and lifestyle and it's impact on PCOS sufferers, is written loud and clear in the pages of this book. You can read life changing stories of recovery from PCOS by those who followed the plan — just a few stories of the many who've found the answer to PCOS through my Healthy Eating and Lifestyle Plan for PCOS. It's been an amazing journey for them and for me. And for so many more who come new to the plan, it's only just beginning.

In this chapter

Volunteers unite for PCOS

Syndrome 'O' versus 'PCOS'

The importance of metabolism in PCOS

Finding out the best foods to eat for PCOS

Other factors

Impact of prescription drugs

Summary

Volunteers unite for PCOS

In 2001, soon after meeting Sasha McDonnell (see page 117 for Sasha's story), I launched diet and lifestyle trials with the help of 100 PCOS volunteers, to understand the impact on PCOS sufferers. This took three years to complete.

Sasha played a key role in helping me by introducing me to PCOS support groups with volunteers willing to take part in the study.

Thousands of women offered to help but it would have been impossible to manage any more than 100 volunteers. Led by the expertise of fertility experts, I needed to familiarise myself with the most common features of PCOS. It was important to focus and concentrate my efforts on what was important, particularly where PCOS symptoms could be reduced through diet, nutrition and exercise.

I used the following criteria to decide who should take part. Volunteers would need to be either:

- Over 35 years old and be desperate to have a baby; or
- Have had unsuccessful IVF treatments; or
- Have three or more symptoms of PCOS; or
- Have been refused IVF; or
- Be obese

'Syndrome O' versus 'PCOS'

One of my PCOS slimmers, 'Rosario', had struggled with weight and other PCOS symptoms for years. Her experience was basically that she had no clarity from doctors or other medical professionals as to what medical condition she was actually suffering from.

This was made worse by the fact that I discovered during the trials with my PCOS volunteers that there was some confusion about what PCOS was actually called. I was often being asked by sufferers to explain the difference between Syndrome O and PCOS. 'Aren't they the same condition?', they'd ask.

Rosario decided to do some research into the difference between the two conditions and uncovered the origin of the term 'Syndrome O'. Here's the answer according to the doctor who coined the term 'Syndrome O': Reproductive Endocrinologist, Dr. Ronald Feinberg.

Syndrome O is a newer name for PCOS. It invokes the dramatic impact of metabolism, genetics, and our changing environment upon the female reproductive system. Since the 1970s, physicians and scientists have been aware of Syndrome X, the metabolic syndrome of insulin overproduction attributed primarily to men. Until recently, little attention was paid to insulin overproduction in women. I conceived the name 'Syndrome O' when I became incensed reading books and articles about 'Syndrome X'. Few Syndrome X experts were making the connection between PCOS and Syndrome X, and the effect of Syndrome X upon women was being ignored.

I eventually described Syndrome O as a triad of understandable problems — Over nourishment (causing insulin overproduction), Ovarian confusion, and Ovulation disruption. These basic problems lead to an array of important women's health issues: abnormal bleeding, missed menses, pregnancy loss, and high-risk pregnancies.

Dr Feinberg maintains that phasing out the designation 'PCOS' should take place because:

- The 'polycysts' seen in women with Syndrome O are not really cysts. They are small underdeveloped follicles that have been induced to grow by the insulin family of hormones

- Most women with PCOS don't have any significant cysts when checked by ultrasound

- Many women with polycystic-appearing ovaries don't have PCOS or Syndrome O. However, there is evidence that some of these women may be at risk of developing Syndrome O

- Syndrome O encompasses a group of women who may ovulate and achieve pregnancy on their own, but then develop insulin-related problems of miscarriage or later pregnancy complications

- Syndrome O invokes the reproductive effects of insulin overproduction on the uterus, placenta, blood vessels, liver, and blood clotting system

- Syndrome O sends a warning message regarding potential health problems to be tested for now and in the future, including diabetes, glucose intolerance (pre-diabetes), lipid abnormalities, and pre-cancerous changes in the uterine lining

The importance of metabolism in PCOS

We've all met those ladies that no matter what they eat, never put on an ounce. That's because they have a naturally fast metabolism (probably just something in their genes) and burn up all the food they eat before it's had a chance to turn into fat. The fact is, the faster your metabolic rate, the more energy you'll use to digest your food; do exercise or just live your life.

The most striking difference between PCOS women and general slimmers is that PCOS women have a sluggish metabolism. I realised by working with my PCOS volunteers that finding ways to increase a sluggish metabolism would be critical to success. I therefore set about analysing all the metabolic rates for each of my volunteers. This would ensure I knew where I was starting from with every individual. Due to insulin resistance, many of my volunteers had uncontrollable cravings for carbohydrates like potatoes, bread, rice pasta and cakes — these will inevitably turn to excess weight and settle in all the usual places, thighs, hips, tums and bums, if improvements in diet and regular exercise don't take place.

I discovered that PCOS sufferers were gaining weight even though they were eating very little. It all fitted together. Because of their sluggish metabolism their digestive system could not burn off carbohydrates as effectively as women with a faster metabolism. This is what was leading to more weight gain. By losing weight healthily and increasing the metabolism with lifestyle changes, plus gentle exercises, the metabolic rate can be improved. This became the focus of all our efforts.

I realised that anything that would boost a sluggish metabolism would go a long way to helping PCOS sufferers. This led me to hit upon the idea that eating small and as often as possible would be the key. I asked our volunteers to eat a tiny amount of vegetable (Nibble™) or protein (Burn™), every 15 minutes (or as often as possible), so they could boost their metabolism regularly and lose more weight. This technique also prevented hunger pangs.

I learned that losing even 3 kg/6 lbs can improve the metabolism which was very inspiring. In 99% of PCOS women the metabolic rate is very slow.

The good news is that it's possible to enjoy food and speed up your metabolism so that you can lose weight and reduce your symptoms. And, if it's your heart's desire, have a much improved chance of becoming pregnant as your hormones begin to level out.

Finding out the best foods to eat for PCOS

Establishing which foods and in which combinations were the most successful for losing weight, and improving the metabolism, was a mammoth task.

My PCOS volunteers spent months trialling diets and undertaking specific tests to ascertain the foods that were most effective for their individual weight loss.

For over 12 months, all 100 volunteers had to be weighed and body measurements taken every week. I had to record in detail how they were feeling on the diets and how successfully they lost weight. The commitment of our volunteers throughout the trials, week in week out, was phenomenal. Without their input this book could never have been written. Thank you ladies!

Other factors

The level of detail I was recording during the trials gave me insights that could not be ignored. For example I found that when my volunteers ate microwaved foods from plastic containers or drank from plastic bottles and other chemical based containers it had a negative impact on weight loss. Across 100 volunteers I was able to determine that due to the hormonal imbalances that accompany PCOS, something as simple as changing from plastic (which leaches chemicals into food and drinks) to glass made a difference to weight loss results. PCOS is a chemical/hormonal imbalance so anything containing chemicals can slow your metabolism further and make weight loss more difficult to achieve.

I came to realise too that the practice for my 'non PCOS' slimmers of eating organic, non-processed foods, that did not contain additives/chemicals was even more important for PCOS women who as we have already established, suffer chemical/hormonal imbalances. Everything natural and fresh was the order of the day.

Impact of prescription drugs

The eight B vitamins — B1, B2, B3, B5, B6, B7, B9, B12 — are essential nutrients that help convert our food into fuel, giving us the energy we need for daily living.

Some PCOS sufferers have to take certain prescription drugs. Some of these medicines can deplete the body of essential B vitamins. Therefore I came to the conclusion that eating good quality, organic animal protein, which is full of B vitamins, is a must.

Summary

After endless hours of testing diets I eventually arrived at a very successful Healthy Eating and Lifestyle Plan for PCOS.

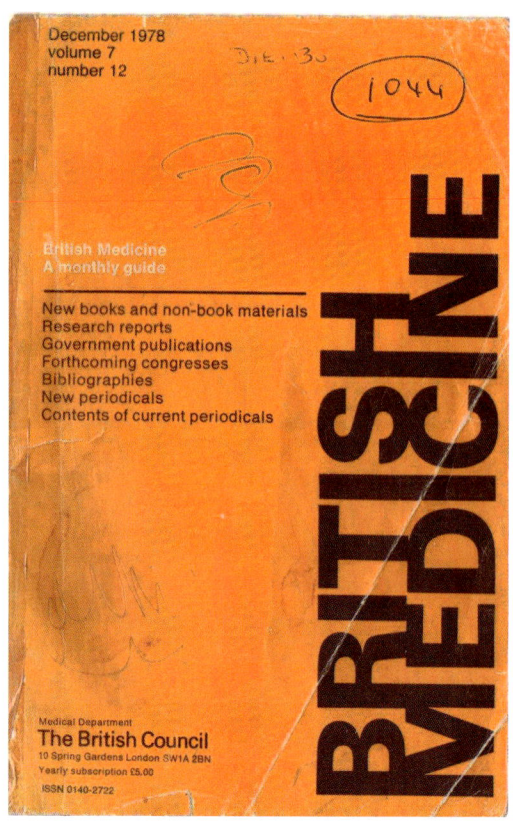

Vitaline, Norah's Healthy Eating and Lifestyle Plan, was included in the British Council British Medicine Guide in 1978.

Many of my PCOS volunteers achieved substantial weight losses during my trials into diet and lifestyle and 97 out of 100 of them became pregnant!

Chapter Three
Fertility

Trying for a baby

More often than not, PCOS causes problems with fertility because the cysts can block the fallopian tubes making it impossible for a woman to ovulate, let alone become pregnant.

For many who desperately want a child of their own, their inability to conceive can be devastating. Too often I see women with PCOS who are quite literally beyond despair in their pursuit of motherhood.

And in an even crueller twist of fate, if they do finally get pregnant by chance or through IVF or other fertility treatments; it's often the case that the cysts can lead to miscarriage. For those of you who have been there, I think you will agree that trying to get pregnant when you have PCOS can be a very rocky road.

The good news is that, one by one, we can remove those rocks from the road. I know this because I have seen how time and time again, women who faithfully follow my Healthy Eating Plan for PCOS can find their cysts shrink after a few weeks. As they start to lose weight and reduce their symptoms they give themselves the best possible chance of becoming more fertile and by extension, increase their chances of pregnancy.

This in turn leads to an improved chance of delivering a baby to full term; without the overwhelming threat of miscarriage.

In addition to following my Healthy Eating and Lifestyle Plan for PCOS, if you are trying for a baby, this chapter gives you some of my best tips to help you increase your chances of becoming pregnant. I hope you'll also be inspired by the 1,000 plus babies who've been born to women who followed my plan.

In this chapter

Ways to improve fertility

Do

Don't

Ways to improve fertility

If you are trying to conceive, why not try these tips; they have worked for others and they could help you.

Female infertility is often caused by a woman's inability to ovulate or release an egg. Failure to ovulate is usually rooted in some hormonal problems. Fortunately, hormonal imbalances are not hard to detect and treatments can be straightforward and relatively effective. Your consultant will be the best person to advise you. However, in many infertility cases, a woman may be producing too little of one hormone or too much of another, such as in the case of PCOS sufferers.

First of all, it is a good idea to work out a pre-conception plan. Most couples don't have sex at the right time and frequency to achieve a pregnancy.

If your periods are regular (28 days from the start of one to the start of another), you should try to have regular intercourse, every other day, if possible, from day 11 to day 17. This is timed from the start of the first day of your last period.

One week before this time of the month, both partners should get plenty of quality sleep, omit alcohol and avoid intercourse altogether, until you reach day 11.

The Menstrual Cycle

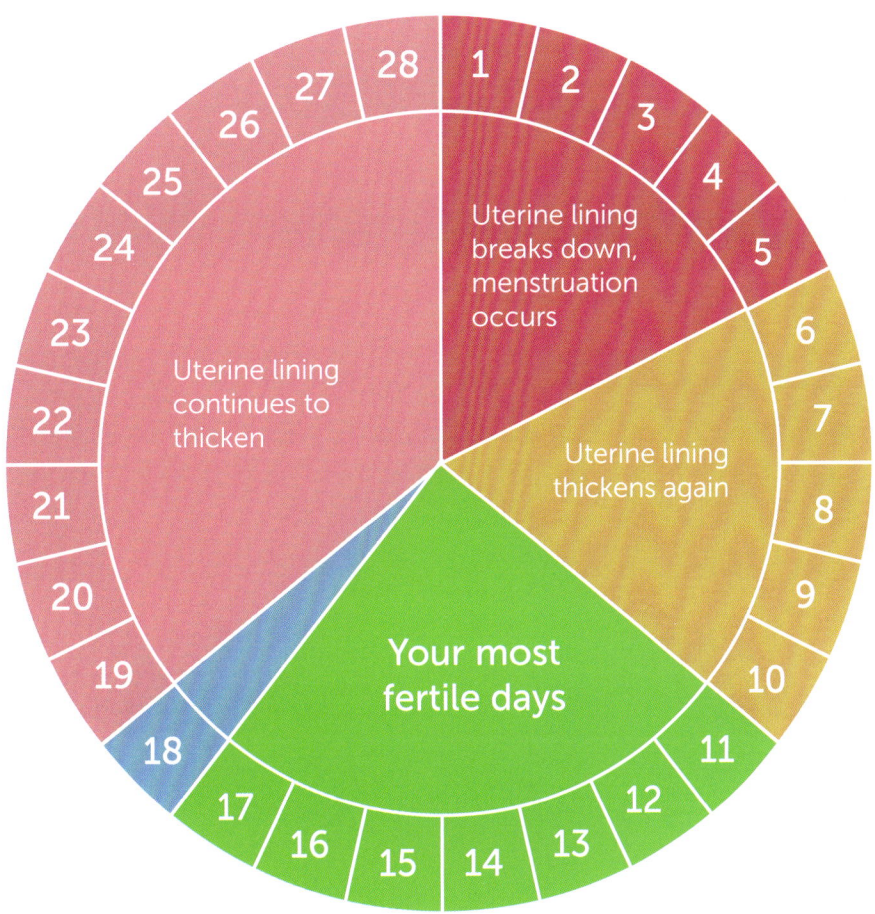

What to do and what not to do

The following have helped to improve the fertility of my clients and will hopefully help you.

Do

- Have a full health check-up (both partners) to make sure that there are no other factors affecting your fertility, such as sperm quality or blockages in the fallopian tubes. It is also important to ensure that you are both immune to rubella (German measles)

- Have more sex, but at the correct time of the month, as stated previously (see fertile days on menstrual cycle diagram on previous page)

- Take time out to relax; **stress** is a huge factor with infertility problems

- Try to relax more, take up yoga or have a relaxing, warm bath before bed. Do not have the water too hot

- Practise deep-breathing exercises to relax

- Sprinkle lavender essence on your pillow at night; it can help some women to relax and get a good night's rest

- Achieving a healthy weight is helpful to fertility for both you and your partner

- Choose fresh organic fruit and vegetables and good organic protein if possible

- Take regular exercise. A good walk every day or a swim can really help

- Drink nettle tea, it can help boost iron levels

- Each night, place a **paper thin** slice of lemon/lime into a cup or mug. Cover with boiling water and let it stand overnight. First thing each morning, drink your now cooled lemon/lime water to detox your digestive system and hydrate your body after a night's sleep NB: DO NOT drink lemon/lime water if you suffer with arthritis

- Drink plenty of filtered or fresh water regularly, in small amounts throughout the day

- Complete your Daily Food Tracker (see page 78); it will help you make sure you are sticking to the right, healthy foods and varying your meals

Don't

- Get obsessed, because stress affects fertility
- Drink coffee or drinks containing caffeine
- Smoke. It is dangerous to your health and can affect fertility
- Drink alcohol or take drugs
- Perform very strenuous exercises
- Drink from cans as they can be lined with aluminium
- Drink from plastic containers or plastic bottles
- Eat processed foods, because they can contain additives, colourings or preservatives. These are chemicals and can affect any chemical/hormonal imbalance you may have
- Drink any fizzy or carbonated drinks
- Miss your meals or go for hours without food — it can reduce sugar levels and lead to bingeing which can undermine your health

'This is a miracle diet plan. I felt better from week two of starting it. I'm more confident because my acne is really clearing up.'
Lillian, Eccles, Greater Manchester, UK

Chapter Four
Our miracle babies

Dreams can come true

In 2002 our first 'miracle baby', Libby McDonnell was born to Sasha and Andy. If you read Sasha and Andy's stories (see pages 117 and 120) you will learn that they spent many years of heartache trying for a baby without success.

Andy and Sasha — proud parents with their little miracle baby, Libby

It wasn't until Sasha followed my Healthy Eating and Lifestyle Plan for PCOS that her and Andy's dream of becoming parents finally came true.

Over the years there have been over 1,000 babies born to my PCOS sufferers. In this chapter you can read about three other women's longed-for miracle babies.

It's been an amazing life affirming experience for me to have been part of their journey to planet Earth. (More miracle stories can be found in the chapter starting on page 115).

In this chapter

Audrey Sheldon and her two miracle sons

Natalie Wilson and her two miracle daughters

Jill Fenske and her miracle son

Audrey Sheldon, Wolverhampton, UK

I didn't really have a period 'til I was about 17, which was also the age when I first got to see a consultant at New Cross Hospital in Wolverhampton about my periods or rather lack of periods.

I had to keep going every six months and keep records of my periods. When I did have a period it would be very heavy and it was always painful. This went on for many years 'til I was about 21 when I had a change of consultant who wanted to do an internal scan and inject dye to check my ovaries, this was when I was told I had PCOS.

Then at my next appointment they told me what they would do next, I was to have an exploration laparoscopy and they would laser the cysts which should help but this didn't happen for another two years. When I did have the operation I was told it had been a success but I overheard a doctor say I'd never have children and that I would always be big. My whole world crashed a lot lot more that day.

As well as irregular periods I also had a battle with my weight. No matter what sort of diet, I could only lose a little, then I would stick again. I have always had a healthy diet but I think people looking at me would think otherwise which also used to get me down.

I told Denn I may have trouble having children

I had already met Denn when I was first diagnosed. I told him from the start I may have trouble having children which didn't bother him, as it was me he wanted. But with this in mind we started trying although we knew it would be hard for me.

Years went by with no luck and still not pregnant, the heartache was unbelievable, but I never felt angry if family or friends had a baby. From the bottom of my heart I was really happy for them and although it wasn't my baby, I would always ask them if I could have a cuddle.

In 1997 we were referred to have fertility treatment called IUI. There was a waiting list for it, so more waiting. In 1999, after seven years together, we finally got married. A few months later we had our first round of IUI fertility treatment but two weeks later my period came.

> 'Every so often I would tell Denn to go and find someone else to have a baby with, which I know annoyed him somewhat. But at the time, I thought it would be for the best.'

We were both devasated

This was our first attempt so we thought maybe next time might be it. The second and third attempts were abandoned because my eggs had matured too far for treatment to continue and would be dangerous to myself.

My fourth and final attempt seemed to go well. Two weeks had gone and nothing so far. But then the pregnancy test at hospital was negative and a few days later my period came.

I was totally devastated. Denn seemed upset but I wasn't sure how he was. Denn wouldn't talk to me and I couldn't help but show how upset I was. Denn seemed to talk OK to my mom, just not me.

> 'But then one day he arrived early from work to tell me he had broken down at work and that he couldn't stop crying. We then cried together, and started sharing our pain and supporting each other.'

A suitable case...if I lost weight!

In 2000 we were referred to the local clinic for IVF. The consultant agreed we were a suitable case for treatment but laid down one condition; I had to lose weight before I would be considered. I knew I was very overweight which wasn't helped from the hormone injections that had sent my weight from 16 stone up to 18 stone.

I asked the consultant what weight I needed to be. When he said 12 ½ stone I could have died there and then. All I could do was to try my best which I knew would be a struggle.

I was just given a leaflet of what not to eat and basically told to get on with it and told to just ring every six months with weight updates.

So I began dieting again and managed to lose 2 stone then like always my weight loss came to a standstill. When I contacted the clinic to tell them how difficult it was I wasn't given any ideas or suggestions.

Norah and Vitaline to the rescue

So in 2003 I gave up dieting but as soon as 2004 came I started again, I wasn't getting any younger so I needed to do something but still my weight wouldn't budge. In July 2005 I had read about a slimming club called Vitaline, which was run by Norah, who helped woman with PCOS lose weight. So I joined online and sent my form and got a diet sheet sent to me and then the weight started to drop off.

After a couple of months on the diet I started to have regular periods which felt odd because I was so used to having one every 12 to 16 months. By the end of October I'd lost a stone and half and was now just over 14 stone so I was getting there for IVF but still had a way to go.

I started to feel different

By this time also, Denn and myself had already come to terms with the fact that we'd never be parents and we should just get on with our life together. But as it happened by the end of December 2005 I started to feel different. My breasts felt different, but I couldn't put my finger on it at the time.

So Christmas came and went and I still had this funny feeling and I said to Denn that I thought I was pregnant, he said 'don't be silly, you can't be'. So the first week in January I bought a pregnancy test and yes that test was positive! I ran downstairs and said; 'I think I am; look', showing him the test. Neither of us could believe it so that week I did five more tests all positive. Believe me I had waited this long, it was hard taking it all in. I had it confirmed at the doctors and slowly it was starting to sink in.

> 'I rang the fertility clinic up and I was so pleased to tell them to take me off the waiting list because I was pregnant! The stunned silence said it all, I don't think they could believe it.'

It was great having my 12 week scan to finally see the tiny baby growing inside, our very long awaited baby. My pregnancy went smoothly and in September 2006, 10 days overdue I was induced. But while in labour, baby's heartbeat kept dropping so I had to have an emergency C-section, a very worrying time for me about baby and Denn had a worrying time with the pair of us. But we had a lovely boy we called Elliott weighing 8 lbs 9 oz.

After a couple of years I went back on Norah's Vitaline diet. I needed to lose the weight again but I wasn't trying for another baby at this point. It wasn't 'til I had been on diet for a year that I said to Denn 'can we try for another baby?'

Although he said 'yes' we weren't like before when we were trying. It was like if it happens it happens, at least we have one little miracle. The second time, it didn't take long, just a couple of months. I was shocked I really didn't expect it to happen so quickly this time but I was so overjoyed.

At around 8 to 9 weeks I started bleeding and really thought I was losing my baby, I couldn't have a scan for another two days after seeing the doctor. I cried all day and couldn't go to work. The day of the scan came and I felt I had lost my baby, I was so nervous going in that room, I couldn't look but then I heard that heartbeat and I cried and looked at the screen and couldn't believe our baby was here, he/she had a strong heartbeat.

Our second little miracle

After the 20 week scan, everything had gone well and I was told I was having a girl .

At the end of my pregnancy, I finally went into labour 12 days late.

I had to have a C-section because labour slowed down when I had my waters broken and they were worried. There we are expecting a girl, when they tell my husband we've had a boy. The midwife left my husband to tell me. I thought he was joking at first. But I was glad I had a healthy baby. It didn't matter they got it wrong. So we had another boy. We called him Noah and he weighed 8 lbs 13 oz, our second little miracle.

> 'I've never met Norah but I have spoken to her and we have emailed each other. She is a lovely person and she has done a wonderful job with helping ladies with PCOS. I'm very grateful to her for her hard work finding a diet for PCOS sufferers that really does work.'

We're so blessed and I can't thank Norah enough for the diet that helped me to have our two beautiful boys. I really am so lucky to have them; my boys that I never thought I would have. I still believe PCOS still has it struggles with the medical profession. More needs to be done to help women.

Audrey wiith her two little miracles; Noah (centre) and Elliott

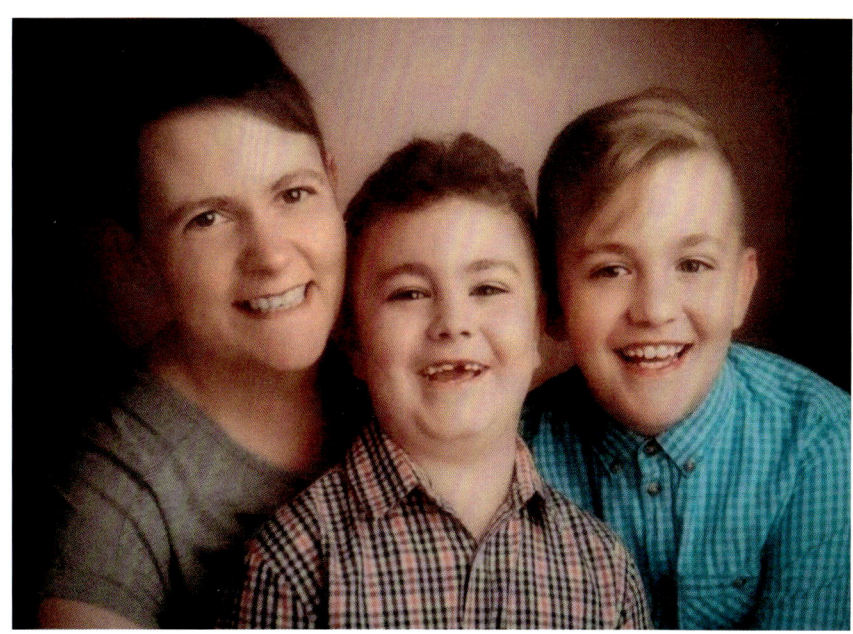

Natalie Wilson, Cheshire, UK

I started with PCOS symptoms from a very early age (16). Being so young and not really understanding what my body was struggling with was very hard. I used to wake every morning and instead of feeling fresh and ready for the day, I felt completely horrid and many times just wanted to stay in bed. I struggled a lot with my mood to the point I thought I was suffering with depression.

In my teens I had battled with my weight. My body would easily gain weight but I found it extremely difficult, if not impossible to lose weight. Because of this ongoing battle I felt I was always on 'a diet' and this ultimately made me completely miserable.

> 'Along with the weight issue, many other PCOS symptoms plagued me every day. Being a young teenage girl, I quickly realised that my excessive hair growth (hirsutism) on my face, neck, chest and other areas was not of the norm. Along with the hair growth I had extremely oily skin and struggled daily with extreme fatigue.'

Eventually after months of living with these awful symptoms I decided to visit my GP with a list of issues I hoped there was a cause for. After discussing at length with my doctor, he was sure I was suffering with some depression and wanted to test for any thyroid problems.

A blood test ruled out any thyroid issues and we were back to square one. I was determined to find out what was wrong with me. After numerous trips back and forth to my GP they finally referred me for some ultrasound scans and a blood test for PCOS.

I wasn't classed as overweight

At the time I had no idea what PCOS was. My doctor explained that; I 'didn't look like the typical PCOS sufferer' as I wasn't classed as being overweight like 'most' PCOS sufferers.

> 'my doctor explained that I 'didn't look like the typical PCOS sufferer.'

After a quick search, I discovered I had almost all of the main symptoms of PCOS and so there was no surprise when the blood test and ultrasound scan showed that indeed I had PCOS.

During this time, I did have further issues with bleeding and so a laparoscopy was performed and I was also diagnosed with endometriosis along with PCOS.

My luck was changing

The few months following this discovery were extremely hard for me. No matter what I tried, medication etc., nothing seemed to keep my symptoms at bay. At this time, my mother and father had recently opened a beauty salon and had told me a lady had joined them who specialises in helping women with PCOS through her miracle diet.

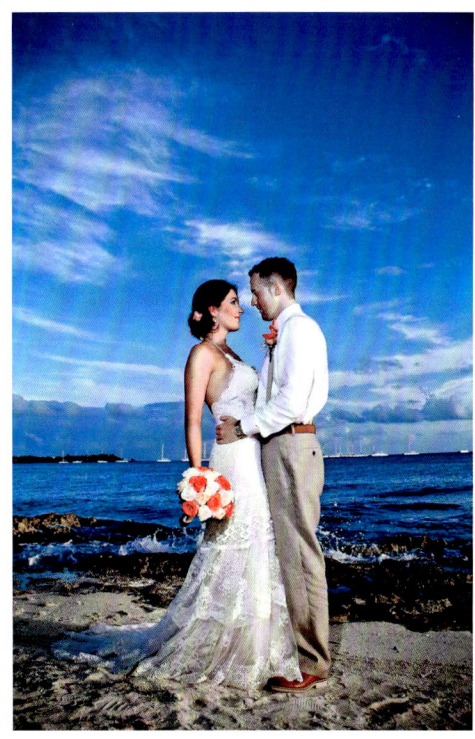

I couldn't believe my luck. I was introduced to Norah and she spent some time with me talking about PCOS and I couldn't believe the information about the condition that I didn't know. Straight away she set me up on a weekly plan.

After a week on Norah's PCOS diet, I couldn't believe the difference. Not only had I lost over 7 lbs in the first week. I finally felt my symptoms were improving. It almost didn't feel real. The diet was so easy to stick to and over the months I managed to lose over 3 stone (just in time for my wedding). I felt great and magically all of my PCOS symptoms had disappeared.

> 'The diet was so easy to stick to and over the months I managed to lose over 3 stone (just in time for my wedding). I felt great and magically all of my PCOS symptoms had disappeared.'

With an eye to the future

As all PCOS sufferers are told, I was worried how my PCOS would affect my chances of conceiving considering how I was told my endometriosis would also make it extremely difficult, if not impossible, to conceive naturally. Norah gave me confidence and explained how the weight loss and diet control will work in my favour for conceiving.

There were lots of hints, tips, and healthy foods to try which Norah explained could help my fertility. Early nights, more sleep, deep breathing exercises, which all helped me to relax. There was an ovulation chart to work through. It all was so useful and helpful.

Annabelle May and Adalynn Eva — my two little miracles

I fell pregnant almost instantly with my precious little girl Annabelle May. It was a true miracle. We couldn't believe our luck and my gynaecology consultant couldn't believe it either.

Our beautiful healthy daughter was born 16 May 2015. I continued to see Norah to keep myself on track and went on to have our second miracle daughter, Adalynn Eva who was born 25th July 2017.

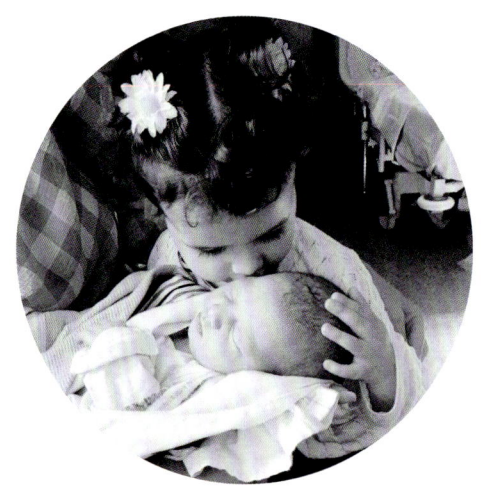

My lucky stars

I count my lucky stars every day that I met Norah. Living with my symptoms was getting unbearable and without Norah's help, I think the road to having children would have been a lot more difficult.

I know exactly what I have to do to keep my PCOS symptoms under wraps. I now live a healthy, happy and symptom free life with my loving husband and beautiful girls.

> 'Norah gave me confidence and explained how the weight loss and diet control will work in my favour for conceiving.'

For any young ladies suffering, and to those who don't necessarily 'fit' the PCOS criteria, there is hope!

When Norah asked if I would like my story in her PCOS book, I was more than happy. If you follow this plan, like I did, there is real hope. Not just losing weight and reducing the devastating symptoms associated with PCOS, but giving yourself the best chance of becoming pregnant and having your own miracle babies. It worked for me.

Thank you Norah!

xxx

Jill Fenske, USA

Jill's a yoga teacher now and weighs less than she did in high school...she says that on my plan she doesn't suffer uncontrollable cravings ever. (Norah)

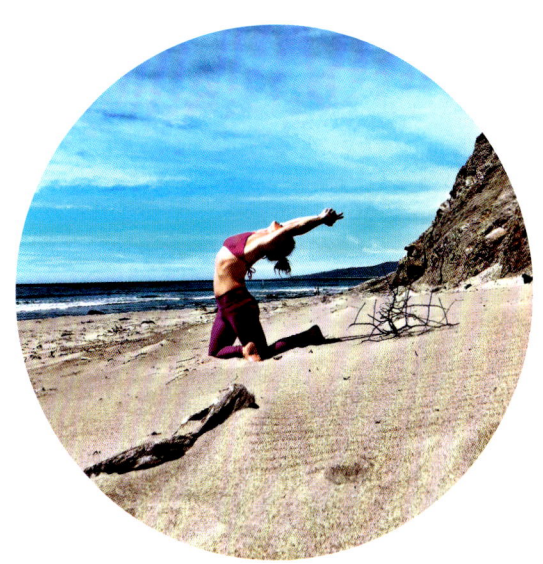

In 2002, my partner and I adopted our first baby. We had always wanted to adopt, and we also knew that at some point I wanted to experience pregnancy and giving birth. So, around 2004, we contacted a fertility specialist to start the process.

I was 32 at the time. I did not have any sense that I would have fertility problems, but being two women, we needed a doctor's help to conceive.

Confirmation of PCOS

The doctor ran a bunch of scans and tests and told me that I had PCOS. He was brusque and did not give me any advice, other than to tell me I was overweight. He just put me on metformin.

I was a retired elite athlete (World Cup Rugby Player) who had allowed myself to go soft after retiring. Granted, I had never been a 'skinny' person — always trying this or that fad diet to bring my weight under control even while in intense training, and nothing had ever worked. I just figured that's how I was made to be.

But by the time 2004 hit I was really unhappy with how my body looked and felt. The metformin actually made me gain more weight, but I figured that was just part of the process of trying to get pregnant.

After trying a few rounds of IUI, a hysteroscopy, and a full hormone workup, the doctor concluded that my uterus was perfectly healthy and while I did have cysts on my ovaries, I did not have any of the other hormonal markers for or symptoms of PCOS. So, I suppose maybe I just had PCO, not the syndrome. They wanted to push me towards IVF, but that was at least $40,000 and they hadn't yet been able to pinpoint what the real problem was.

SO...I decided, finally, to do some research and take matters into my own hands. And to switch doctors. His bedside manner was horrible and he was SO unhelpful through the first part of our process.

Research led me to Norah and her Vitaline team

I did some research online and found out that women who had PCOS had the most luck getting pregnant when they lost weight. Ugh. I had been down that road before, I thought, and I knew that was going to be very hard to do.

Then I landed on Norah Cozens and Vitaline. It wasn't a huge organization, but it was specific to what I needed.

It was the nibbles and burns that got me through. This was, BY FAR, the easiest diet to stick to EVER. I was never hungry. And I wasn't an angel, either. Sometimes a little lick of the frosting spatula here, or an extra glass of wine there…and because I wasn't an angel, the weight didn't come off super fast. But it came off. Slowly, one week at a time, it came off.

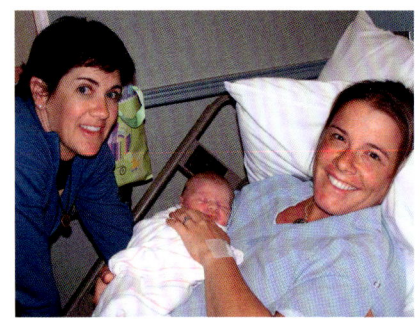

Proud parents, Kelly and Jill are clearly thrilled by the arrival of their newborn son, Reese

Time to change Doctors

Norah had told me that 25 lbs seemed to be the magic number, so when I got close to losing 25 lbs (I started at 175), I started looking for a new fertility doctor. My periods still weren't super regular, but I had been seeing an acupuncturist and they were at least coming every 32-45 days.

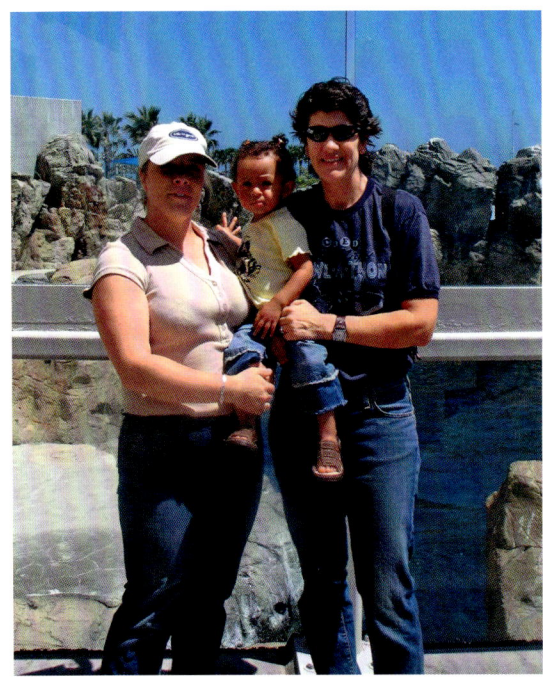

Jill, Shannon and Kelly before Jill found Norah

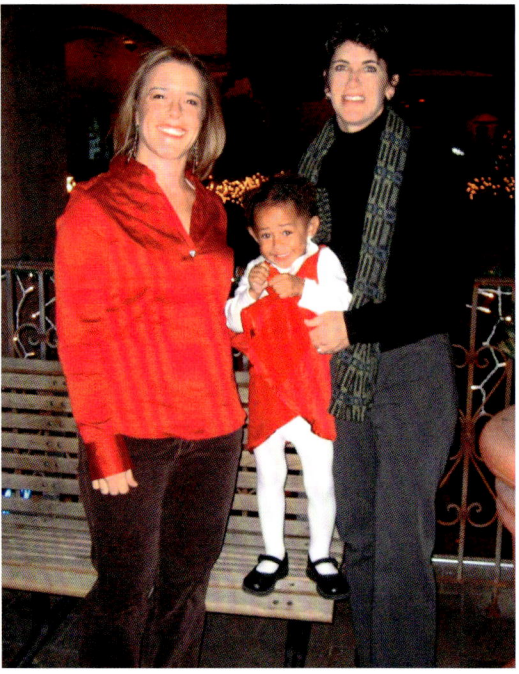

After finding Norah

When I found the doctor, he was skeptical that doing IUI would work, but he listened to what I had been through and was willing to try. He followed my ovulation via ultrasound and when I got to day 21 and still hadn't ovulated, he was starting to make sounds like this wasn't going to happen this cycle. I asked for his patience.

> 'A couple of days later the egg matured and we inseminated. I conceived on that very first try, after having followed Norah's programe for almost a year.'

Our miracle baby arrives

Our beautiful and strong baby boy was born in July of 2006. I used Norah's program during my pregnancy when my doctor told me I was gaining weight a little too fast, and then after giving birth in order to lose the baby weight. I have kept it off and then some. Today (May 2018) I am at 135 lbs, with a strong athletic body. I still mostly eat the way Norah taught me to eat — it is what works best for my body.

And I don't really miss the foods that I avoid. I allow myself to have them when I want them, but I find that I don't really want them that much. The cycle of uncontrollable craving has long since been broken.

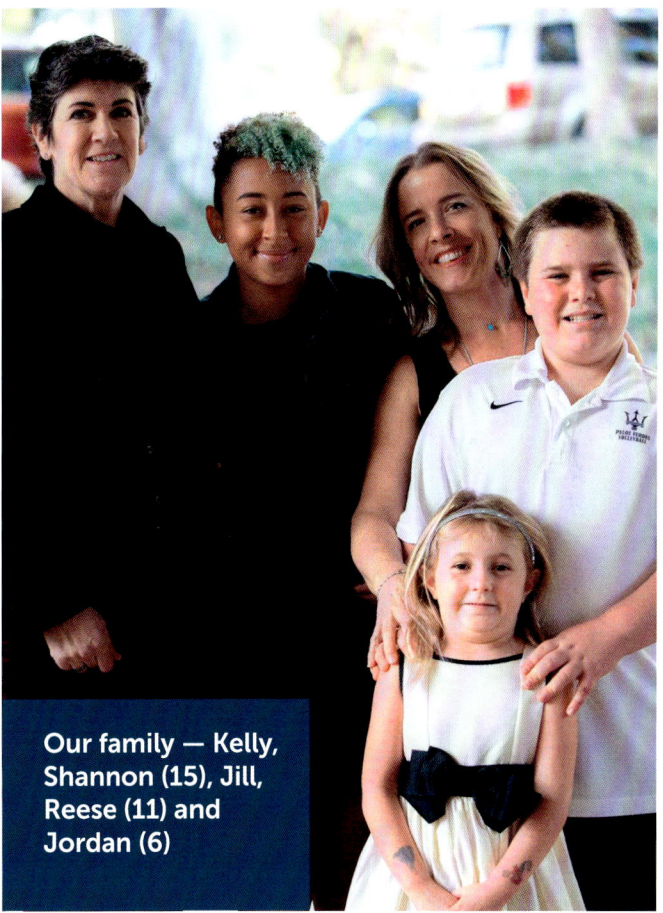

Our family — Kelly, Shannon (15), Jill, Reese (11) and Jordan (6)

I cannot thank Norah enough; she was a Godsend to me and my family.

You are amazing, thank you Norah!

Chapter Five
Medical info

Understanding PCOS

If you suffer with Polycystic Ovary Syndrome (PCOS) you'll probably want to understand a little bit more about how it sits within a medical context.

In this chapter, I provide a very basic overview, written in layman's terms of PCOS and PCO (polycystic ovaries but without the symptoms of the syndrome) to help you understand the difference between them.

In this chapter

Female reproductive system

PCOS symptoms and PCO

Diagnosis, prevention and treatment

Non-cancerous ovarian cysts

Female reproductive system

To understand what is happening in a polycystic ovary it is necessary to explain how ovaries normally work and how the hormones they produce cause the monthly cycle of bleeding and egg release, known as the menstrual cycle.

First let's take a look at the female reproductive system so we can 'see' where ovarian cysts are located.

Your reproductive system consists of two walnut-sized ovaries located on either side of the uterus. They are nestled under the fringed ends of the fallopian, or uterine tubes. These tubes create a pathway for a released egg to reach the centre of the uterus (the womb).

Many women will have cysts at some point during their childbearing years. Most are completely without symptoms. However, some types of ovarian cysts can cause serious health problems.

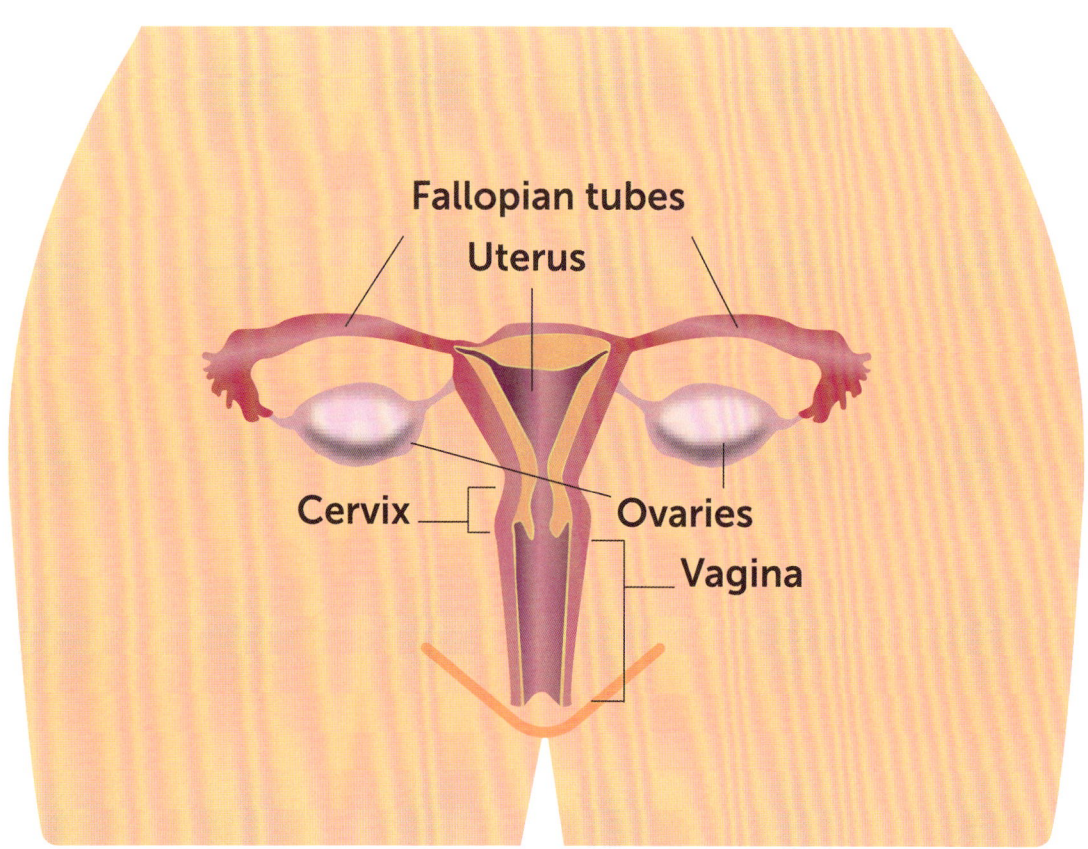

An ovarian cyst is a fluid-filled sac usually found on the surface of an ovary. There are many types of ovarian cysts, each with a different underlying cause.

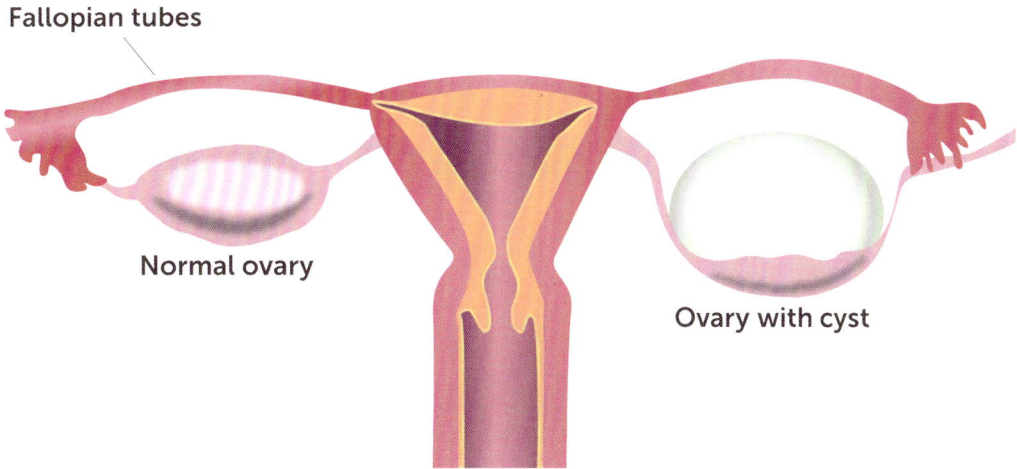

The Menstrual Cycle

During the menstrual cycle, one ovary will develop and mature an egg. The egg is encased in a sac called a follicle. Around day 14 of the menstrual cycle, ovulation occurs and the egg is released from the ovary.

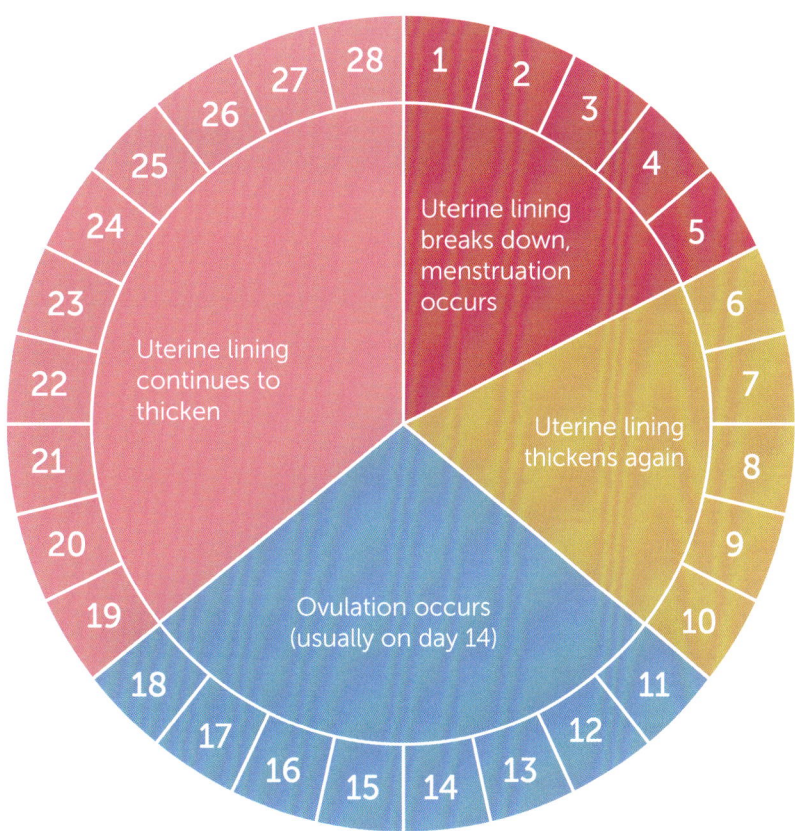

PCOS symptoms and PCO

Polycystic Ovary Syndrome (PCOS)

During the diet and lifestyle trials undertaken by 100 PCOS volunteers; with support from medical professionals; I learned that every PCOS sufferer may have at least one or more of the many PCOS symptoms.

For example, some suffered severely from two or three symptoms while others suffered many of the symptoms, but only mildly. This is the reason why PCOS is difficult to diagnose.

If you have been diagnosed with PCOS this means you have one or more symptoms of PCOS and a scan has revealed cysts on your ovaries.

Symptoms of PCOS

- Hirsutism (excessive facial and/or bodily hair)
- Thinning hair
- Acne/oily skin
- Irregular menstrual cycles (which may lead to infertility)
- Infertility
- Ovulation problems
- Recurring miscarriages
- Hormonal imbalances
- Irregular, non-existent or flooding periods
- Insulin resistance
- A slow or sluggish metabolism
- Weight gain (which can lead to obesity)
- Cravings or binges on carbohydrates or sugary foods
- Extreme fatigue, aching joints
- Stress, depression and mood swings
- Skin tags and brown skin patches
- Pelvic pain – a dull ache, either constant or intermittent, possibly radiating to the lower back or thighs
- Pelvic pain during intercourse

- Pelvic pain just before your period begins or just after it ends
- A fullness or heaviness in your abdomen
- Feeling of pressure on your bladder or rectum
- Nausea or breast tenderness
- Creamy or clear egg white-like vaginal discharge that persists unchanged for a month or more

> **NOTE: If you have any of the following symptoms you should see your doctor/other health professional as soon as possible.**
>
> **If you have sudden, severe or spasmodic pain in your lower abdomen, especially if accompanied by fever, vomiting, or signs of shock (cold, clammy skin, rapid breathing, weakness), go immediately to the emergency department of the nearest hospital.**

Wider health problems of PCOS

If PCOS is not managed through a healthy diet, making appropriate lifestyle changes and following a sensible exercise programme, far more serious health problems can occur such as:

- High blood pressure
- Heart conditions
- Diabetes
- Bone density problems (many older PCOS sufferers have hip problems requiring hip replacements)
- Strokes
- Lack of periods can cause problems with the cervix
- Not shedding the lining of the womb regularly (irregular or no periods)
- Cancer of the womb lining (endometrial cancer)

Polycystic Ovaries (PCO)

A woman may have polycystic ovaries but none of the signs or symptoms that make up the syndrome. Most of these women will have a regular menstrual cycle and then discover they have PCO during a scan.

Around 20% of the female population has PCO, many of whom may never know they have it.

In conclusion

It is not entirely clear why some women will manage to stay symptom free (PCO) while others seem to have every symptom or are badly affected by one in particular (PCOS).

It seems very likely that PCOS is an inherited condition, although the gene or group of genes responsible have not yet been found. Although it may well be that a combination of inherited genes determine your symptoms. **One of the main factors influencing symptoms is excess weight.**

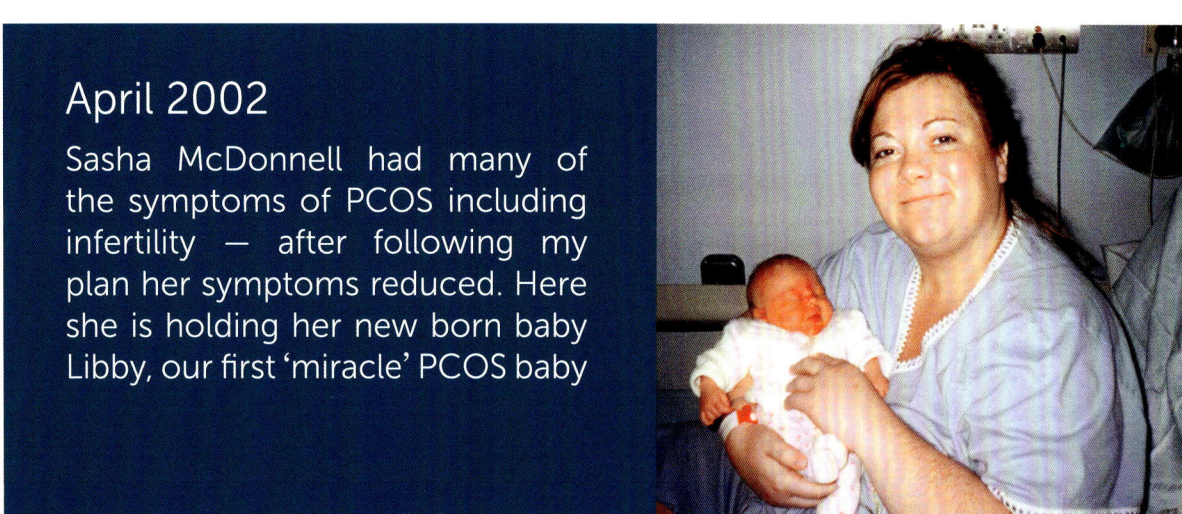

April 2002

Sasha McDonnell had many of the symptoms of PCOS including infertility — after following my plan her symptoms reduced. Here she is holding her new born baby Libby, our first 'miracle' PCOS baby

Diagnosis, prevention and treatment

Diagnosing ovarian cysts

Pelvic exam
An ovarian cyst may be discovered by your doctor during a pelvic examination. If a cyst is suspected, an ultrasound is usually the next step.

Pelvic ultrasound
Ultrasound is a painless procedure where sound waves are transmitted through your pelvic area and an image of your ovaries and uterus is shown on a video screen. The image is analysed to determine the nature of the cyst.

Laparoscopy
Laparoscopy is a surgical procedure involving a thin, lighted telescope which is inserted through a small incision into the abdomen.

Can ovarian cysts be prevented?

It may not be possible to completely prevent ovarian cysts. However, it is possible to minimize the probability that they will form and grow.

You can do this in several ways:

- Improve the quality of your diet (my Healthy Eating and Lifestyle Plan for PCOS is designed to do this)
- Increase your exercise (follow my daily exercise regime on page 108)
- Control chronic stress (yoga, meditation and practising mindfulness can all help with your stress levels. Being well organised and making sure you make time for yourself is a stress buster too)

Treating ovarian cysts

Watchful waiting
If you have no symptoms and an ultrasound scan shows a small, fluid-filled cyst, don't be surprised if your doctor simply schedules another pelvic exam and ultrasound in a few weeks' time.

The concept behind 'watchful waiting' is not to actively treat the cyst, waiting instead until it does not go away as your hormones change. A changing or growing cystic ovary needs further investigation.

If you have a functional cyst that is large in size and causing some symptoms, birth control pills may be prescribed. The purpose of birth control pills is to alter your hormone levels so the cyst will shrink. Birth control pills can also reduce the probability of other cysts growing.

Surgery

Your cyst may be surgically removed if it is large, solid or filled with debris, persistently growing, irregularly shaped, or causing pain or other symptoms. If the cyst is not cancerous, it can be surgically removed without also removing the ovary. This is called a cystectomy. In some cases, the doctor may want to remove the affected ovary, while leaving the other intact in order to maintain your ability to have a normal hormone cycle.

Are ovarian cysts dangerous?

Most ovarian cysts are harmless 'functional' or 'physiologic' cysts.

Multiple ovarian cysts are one hallmark of PCOS. The hormonal disruptions that accompany PCOS can result in persistent acne, excessive bodily hair, thinning scalp hair, infertility, obesity, and an increased risk of diabetes, cardiovascular disease, and uterine or breast cancer.

Ovarian cysts can cause discomfort during intercourse. They may bleed, rupture, or twist the ovary, causing significant pelvic pain.

Sudden or severe pelvic pain, especially with vomiting or a fever, should be treated as a medical emergency. Some ovarian cysts can become cancerous. These are all rare cancers and are most common in women in their 50s. Cancerous ovaries are usually not painful unless they grow very large before they are discovered.

Annual pelvic exams are the best preventative method for detecting gynaecological cancers in the early, most treatable stages.

Non-cancerous ovarian cysts

Functional (physiologic) cysts

The most common type of ovarian cyst is the functional cyst, also called a physiologic cyst. 'Physiologic' means the cyst is not caused by a bacteria or virus. It develops from tissue that changes during the process of ovulation. Your ovaries normally grow cystic structures called follicles each month. Typically, these revert back to normal ovarian tissue after ovulation. But sometimes there is a glitch and the fluid-filled cyst stays on for a while. There are two types of functional cysts:

1 Follicular cyst

Normally, during the menstrual cycle, the egg is released from the follicle and travels down the fallopian tube where it may then become fertilized by a sperm cell. This happens when the pituitary gland in your brain sends a message, by increasing luteinizing hormone (LH), to the follicle holding the ripening egg. This is called a 'LH surge'. If the LH surge does not occur, the follicle doesn't rupture or release its egg. Instead, it grows until it becomes a cyst. These cysts seldom cause pain, are usually harmless, and may disappear within two or three menstrual cycles.

2 Corpus luteum cyst

When there is a successful LH surge and the egg is released, the follicle responds by becoming a new, temporary little secretory gland called the corpus luteum. The corpus luteum produces large amounts of progesterone and a little bit of oestrogen, to prepare the uterus for conception.

But occasionally, after the egg is released, the escape hatch seals off prematurely and tissue accumulates inside, causing the corpus luteum to enlarge. This type of cyst will usually disappear after a few weeks. Rarely, a corpus luteum cyst can grow to 7.5-10 cm/3"- 4" in diameter and potentially bleed into itself, or twist your ovary, thus causing pelvic or abdominal pain.

Other types of cysts

Dermoid cyst

A dermoid cyst is mainly fat but can also contain a mix of different tissues. They are often small and usually don't cause symptoms. Very rarely, they become large and rupture, causing bleeding into the abdomen, which is a medical emergency.

Endometrioma or 'chocolate cyst'

These are cysts that form when endometrial tissue (the type that lines the inside of the uterus) invades an ovary. It is responsive to monthly hormonal changes, which causes the cyst to fill with blood. It's called a 'chocolate cyst' because the blood is a dark, reddish-brown colour.

Multiple endometriomas are found in the condition called 'endometriosis'. Although often asymptomatic, chocolate cysts can be painful, especially during your period or during intercourse.

Cystadenoma

Cystadenomas are cysts that develop from cells on the surface of your ovary. They are usually benign. Occasionally, they can become quite large and thus interfere with abdominal organs and cause pain.

Multiple cysts – the polycystic ovary

Women who don't ovulate on a regular basis can develop multiple cysts. The ovaries are often enlarged and contain many small cysts, clustered under a thickened, outer capsule. There are many factors that cause a woman to not ovulate and develop polycystic ovaries. PCOS is a complex condition that involves multiple hormonal and organ system dysfunction. Multiple ovarian cysts are just one facet of this disorder.

Chapter Six
Before you start

Preparing for the 'new you'

Before you start my Healthy Eating and Lifestyle Plan for PCOS, I recommend you have a good read through this chapter.

It contains lots of hints and tips to ease the journey, and set you off on the right foot as you begin on your road to recovery from PCOS and the start of the 'new you'.

> **In this chapter**
>
> Some Frequently Asked Questions about the plan
> A Guide to a 'good' day
> More tips to help you succeed
> Your Sample Daily Food Tracker
> What to do if you are constipated
> Healthy habits to adopt

'I was 5' tall, 13 stone and 7 lbs and hairy. Agonising periods one month, then nothing for several months, were destroying my life. I could not socialize for fear of starting my unexpected, flooding period.

'On the PCOS Healthy Eating Plan, I lost four stone in six months. I have kept my weight off for over six years now. My PCOS symptoms have diminished, my bodily hair has gone and my periods are regular and manageable. Thank you!'

Joan, Wales

Frequently asked questions about my plan

How long does it take to lose weight on your plan?

If you have more than 19 kg/42 lbs to lose; you can generally expect to lose between 4.5-6kg/10-14 lbs on the plan over a period of four weeks. Some people lose more depending on their commitment, self-discipline and how much weight they have to lose.

Along with varying your food regularly and incorporating the recommended daily lifestyle practices in my plan, you can continue to lose weight. If the guidance is strictly followed you can expect to lose approximately 1 kg/2 lbs per week. Doctors do not recommend losing weight any faster than this as 'crash dieting' i.e., losing weight too fast, can result in muscle loss instead of fat loss.

What is your Healthy Eating and Lifestyle Plan for PCOS?

It is a healthy low fat, low carbohydrate diet that uses only fresh food and includes good quality animal protein, fresh fruit and vegetables.

Combined with a healthy lifestyle and very easy daily exercises (see page 108) and other beneficial practices such as eating little and often, but very healthily, you will never be hungry on this diet.

Key points to note

- **You must eat to lose weight**
- **You will be eating much more than usual but you will be eating healthily**
- **You will never be hungry on this plan (unless you have an extraordinarily large appetite)**

What are the daily practices it teaches?

My Binge Recovery Guide

Before you even get started on my plan; it is important to address the big problem of binge eating. It is a common problem for slimmers and it's a psychological barrier to successful weight loss; as it can be so overwhelming. Bingeing can prevent people from even starting on a weight reduction plan.

Recognising you have a problem with binge eating is essential. Knowing what to do about it is another matter.

But do not despair; I have devised and tried and tested my Binge Recovery Guide for daily use, if necessary. It depends how big a problem bingeing poses for you.

It is popular among my slimmers and has helped them immeasurably in diverting and managing bingeing successfully. It can help you identify your binge triggers and suggests ways of managing them so that eventually, with daily practise, you *can* win the battle of the binge and stop bingeing forever! (See page 29 for my Binge Recovery Guide).

Real food only

Because of the hormonal and chemical imbalances that accompany PCOS, I recommend eating **only fresh 'real' food;** preferably organic. Organic food is nutrient rich and exactly how nature intended us to eat. Processed food is inevitably full of chemicals; a definite 'no-no' if you have PCOS. Avoid eating gum too, it fills you full of wind and makes you hungry.

Eat organic

Organic food has far less additives and/or pesticides than non-organic food. This is very important when it comes to PCOS sufferers because, as part of this condition they have hormonal/chemical imbalances.

I know buying organic can be more expensive but it's extremely important on my plan. I hope you will see it as an investment in your health. But if you cannot afford organic every day then at least try and eat organic once a week.

Eat three fruits a day

Eating three pieces of fruit a day will help to nourish you. Kiwis and pears are vitamin rich and are always the best choice. Eating berries and seeds with breakfast cereals and salads is another great source of vitamins. Avoid bananas and cherries; although they are good for you, they are best eaten only after you have reached your desired weight, as they take longer than other fruits to burn off.

Eat fresh vegetables

Make sure you eat lots of leafy green vegetables with your meals. Vegetables can also be made into soup and eaten before any main meal or salad. Eat some hot soup or have a hot drink before eating cold food such as salad. Avoid cooked root vegetables like carrots.

Avoid starchy foods

Until you have reached your target weight, it is important that you reduce your intake of starchy foods like bread, and potatoes; but avoid pasta and rice altogether. PCOS sufferers struggle to burn these foods off because they can be insulin resistant and carbohydrate sensitive.

Once you have increased your metabolism and reached your desired weight, you can reintroduce these foods into your diet in moderation. But please note that keeping certain carbohydrates i.e., pasta and rice, to a minimum, is essential to the ongoing management of your PCOS symptoms.

Avoid salt

It is important for PCOS sufferers to avoid all chemicals. That's why you should reduce your salt intake as much as possible. Never sprinkle salt on food. Cut down or avoid the use of salt in cooking as salt causes water retention problems. If it is not possible for you to omit salt, try using products like sea salt or lo-salt. Why not use herbs to flavour your food?

Avoid smoked food

It is important to avoid smoked, salty or spicy foods which contain salt. Smoked food can be salt cured and can cause the body to hold unnecessary fluids. Too much salt or smoked foods can result in high blood pressure as well as water retention.

Eating every 15 minutes

For over 40 years I have recommended eating a tiny piece of vegetable or protein every 15 minutes throughout the day and evening, or whenever you can. That's because regularly eating such a small amount keeps your metabolism boosted. It also bombards your body with essential vitamins throughout the day and stops hunger pangs.

This patented system is known as Nibbles™ (vegetables) and Burns™ (proteins). It is an essential part of your daily routine on my Healthy Eating and Lifestyle Plan for PCOS. If you do not adopt this daily practise, your weight loss success will take much, much longer to achieve. Losing weight too slowly while at the same time battling binge eating is a major barrier to success for all slimmers. It can lead to demotivation and make it much harder to stay on track.

Eat hot food

Hot food is preferable for keeping your metabolism working. If you are having a salad or anything cold, like a sandwich, it's a good idea to have either a hot drink or a bowl of soup beforehand.

Vary your food

It's important to vary your food. Doing so will make sure that you nourish yourself with a wide range of nutrients and essential vitamins while at the same time 'firing up' your metabolism.

Morning and afternoon snacks

Don't miss your morning and afternoon snacks – they make sure your metabolism keeps working until your next meal and ensure you don't get hungry.

Daily lemon or lime water – keeping hydrated

Hydrating your body after a night's sleep is very important because it's at night when the body is busy repairing itself.

It is also important to keep hydrating your body throughout the day. It helps with weight loss and PCOS symptom reduction as fluids are essential to helping your body eradicate unwanted chemicals. It can also help with constipation problems and is a great detox as well as being good for your skin.

I recommend you prepare a **paper thin** slice of lemon or lime each evening and place it in a mug or a cup. Top it up with hot water and let it stand on your bedside cabinet overnight or for at least four hours. This enables vitamins in the lemon and lime to mix with the water so that in the morning, when you drink it (preferably before your very easy daily exercises – some of which you can do in bed); you will rehydrate your system after a night's sleep and give yourself a vitamin boost.

If you can taste the lemon or lime in your water you have sliced it too thickly. It should be **paper thin**.

Please note: If you suffer from arthritis you should not drink lemon or lime water; just drink plain, boiled, cooled water.

Other drinks

You can keep topping up your lemon or lime water with hot water throughout the day and you can also drink teas and coffees but try and choose decaffeinated drinks – they do not impact on your mood and will help you sleep better. Avoid any kind of cordial because the sugar content is generally too high. Any low-calorie drink is fine and of course plain, still water.

If you have problems sleeping, camomile tea at night can help.

Alcohol

After you have completed the first week on the diet; you can, have a glass of red wine every day. Red wine contains bioflavanoids which can help protect the heart.

Please note: I recommend you drink responsibly. You should seek medical advice before drinking alcohol, particularly if you have a medical condition that could be adversely affected by alcohol.

Avoiding processed foods

Processed foods are generally full of preservatives. Given that we are trying to avoid additives and chemicals so that we can help redress hormonal imbalances in PCOS sufferers, it stands to reason that I do not recommend processed foods at all.

A sweet tooth?

Make up some sugar free jelly in advance and keep it in the fridge. That way, if you find yourself hankering after something sweet you can satisfy your sweet tooth without going off the rails. But avoid products containing sorbitol, or OSEs ie: dextrOSE, lactOSE, fructOSE and glucOSE as these are all forms of sugar.

Constipation

Being constipated is something that you need to pay attention to in order to help maintain a healthy system. If you are constipated it's a good idea to get 'going' with hot Pear and Prunes before bed at night (see remedy on page 79). The major cause of constipation is not drinking enough liquid, not eating enough leafy green vegetables and a lack of exercise. Drink plenty of plain water too.

Very easy 5-minute daily exercises

Being physically active (along with eating healthily) is essential to good health. There are hundreds of exercise regimes circling the planet, either online or on DVD; and some of them are quite extreme. The problem is that if you are overweight; some exercises can be physically impossible.

I recommend a series of **very easy** daily exercises that have been designed by a professional trainer (see page 108 for the exercises). They are meant to be done very slowly and comfortably and can help you tone up as you lose weight as well as speed up your metabolism.

Eating some protein just before bed

I recommend eating a small amount of protein just before bed as this keeps your metabolism working for a while, after you fall asleep — this could be a dessert spoon of cottage cheese or a stock cube sized piece of protein such as chicken or beef.

Exfoliating daily

Every time you shower or bathe, exfoliate by brushing the skin — I have added 'exfoliating mitts' to your shopping list on page 86 as these are easy to use and not expensive. Exfoliating can help improve your circulation, reduce unwanted fluids and tone your skin. You can even gently exfoliate your face to improve skin tone.

Daily Food Tracker

It is important to keep a food diary. Slimmers who keep track of what they are eating daily are more successful at losing weight (see page 78 for your Sample Daily Food Tracker).

The Maintenance Diet

Once you have reached your target weight you should go on to the Maintenance Diet (see page 139). If you stick to the guidance in this additional healthy eating plan and limit the number of treats you enjoy, you will be able to maintain your weight. You will also continue to eat healthy, delicious food on this plan and can look forward to — **no more yo-yo dieting!**

Getting a hobby

If you don't already have a hobby it is a very good idea to get one. If you busy yourself with a hobby it can help to stop you thinking about food.

Guide to a 'good' day

These tips will help you to achieve maximum weight loss:

- Each evening make up some lemon or lime water. Take a **paper thin** slice of lemon or lime, place in a mug or cup, fill with boiling water, leave overnight to cool and drink first thing every morning – this will cleanse and hydrate your system. If you suffer from arthritis do not drink lemon or lime water; just have plain, boiled and cooled water

- After your lemon/lime water – do your daily exercises as set out on page 108

- Do not miss breakfast (choose from the selection of breakfasts on page 103)

- Start your Nibbles™ imediately after breakfast. Pack in as many as you can during the course of the day and evening eating one every 15 minutes to boost your metabolism (see page 91 for information on Nibbles™)

- Eat your mid-morning snack

- Do not miss lunch (choose from the selection of lunches on page 105)

- Eat your mid-afternoon snack

- Do not miss your evening meal (choose from the selection on page 107)

- Do your very easy, gentle exercises before bed (page 108)

- Eat your last portion of protein such as chicken, fish, beef, pork, just before bed (about the size of a stock cube or choose a dessert spoon of cottage cheese)

- DO NOT miss any meals – it will slow down your metabolism

- As a PCOS sufferer it's important to substitute bread for crispbread or yeast free bread

> 'The road to success is dotted with many tempting parking places.'
> —**Unknown**

> 'The journey of 1,000 miles starts with one step.'
> — **Lao Tzu**

> 'Believe you can and you're halfway there.'
> —**T. Roosevelt**

More tips to improve weight loss

- Vary your food – it will improve your weight loss
- Be sure to sprinkle 10 berries and a ¼ teaspoon of seeds on your breakfast cereals. Alternatively, sprinkle your seeds on salads or soups
- Don't miss your morning and afternoon snacks; they make sure your metabolism keeps working until your next meal
- Eat hot food or have a hot drink or hot soup, before eating cold food
- Make up sugar free jelly and keep it in the fridge – it will satisfy a sweet tooth when you need something sweet
- If you feel hungry, eat a small amount of protein, such as a spoonful of cottage cheese or drink a hot cup of homemade soup if you feel hungry – this will keep you going until your next meal
- Using your exfoliating mitts to exfoliate every time you shower or bathe by rubbing your 'problem areas'; usually hips, tummy and bottom gently, until your skin is slightly pink — then stop rubbing. This can help improve your circulation and make your skin feel soft and smooth. Be sure to moisturise after drying yourself
- Keep a note of what you eat every day — slimmers who write down what they eat tend to achieve better weight losses because they are consciously aware of what they are eating (see page 78 for your Daily Food Tracker — type this up and use it every day!)
- Avoid starches and carbohydrates at night – you don't have enough time to burn them off before bed
- Avoid foods containing sorbitol or OSEs like fructOSE or glucOSE, for example. They are not healthy
- Avoid chewing gum. It fills you full of wind and makes you hungry
- Eat 'Pear and Prunes' for constipation (see remedy on page 79)
- Your Nibbles™ or Burns™ are the secret to your success – even a few daily will help
- Measure yourself regularly to note your inch/centimetre loss. Be sure to record your measurements on your Daily Food Tracker (see page 78 for a sample)
- Do your daily exercises (see page 108) — exercise tones up your body and diet loses your weight!
- Remember – 'a minute in the mouth is a month on the hips'
- Get a hobby – it will take your mind off food! Preferably something active

> 'Ask yourself if what you're doing today will get you closer to where you want to be tomorrow.'
> —Anonymous

Your Sample Daily Food Tracker

Complete your food tracker EVERY DAY (see a 3-day sample below). Type up a full 7-day version. It will help you keep track of what you are eating so that you can improve your chances of having a good weight loss, week by week.

Name:		Date:	

Ideal Weight:		Weight at start of week:		Weight at end of week:	

Measurements:					
Bust:	Waist:	Tummy:	Hips:	Tops of arms:	Tops of legs:

	Nibbles™ (Which type)	Bladder movement (Indicate with a √ each time you have one)	Bowel movement (Indicate with a X each time you have one)
DAY 1			
Breakfast			
Mid-morning snack			
Lunch			
Mid-afternoon snack			
Evening Meal			
Supper			
Small amount of protein before bed			
DAY 2			
Breakfast			
Mid-morning snack			
Lunch			
Mid-afternoon snack			
Evening Meal			
Supper			
Small amount of protein before bed			
DAY 3			
Breakfast			
Mid-morning snack			
Lunch			
Mid-afternoon snack			
Evening Meal			
Supper			
Small amount of protein before bed			

Please indicate the number and type of Nibbles™ eaten in the week ....

What to do if you are constipated

> **IMPORTANT:** It is not essential that you have a daily bowel movement. On my Healthy Eating and Lifestyle Plan for PCOS, there is very little wastage. You are not eating large amounts of bread or other stodgy foods; therefore, you are not making the bulk so you may not have a bowel movement each day.

As long as you are feeling well whilst you are losing weight and are generally healthy, you are probably not constipated.

However, sometimes when you are on a diet plan or change the type of food you are eating, you may feel constipated. Certain medications can also make you feel constipated. In many cases this can be resolved by drinking more fluids, especially water; eating more leafy, green vegetables and fresh fruit and taking more exercise. If after trying all of these you still feel constipated, the following tried and tested remedy can help.

Pear and prune remedy

Take a large pear, including the skin, chop into small cubes and place in a bowl. Be sure to remove the stone in the prunes. Cover with water, add four prunes and then microwave for two minutes until the pear is 'mushy'. You can also heat the pears and prunes in a pan and simmer for a couple of minutes if you do not have a microwave.

> *'Food should be our medicine and our medicine should be our food.'*
> — **Hippocrates**

Eat the pear and prune mixture and drink the juice, as hot as possible, just before bedtime. It's important that this remedy is performed before bed as the bowel needs to be relaxed for this to work effectively during the night.

The fibre from the pear and prunes will act on the bowel while you are asleep. The hot fluid will lubricate the bowel during the night and within one hour of drinking your lemon water in the morning, you should have the desired effect. If your bowels are very stubborn, try this each night until you get the desired results.

Healthy habits to adopt

Not all PCOS sufferers have weight problems, but all can gain the benefits of healthy eating. Your diet can increase your metabolism, and you should start to feel healthier after the first few weeks on my Healthy Eating and Lifestyle Plan for PCOS.

As you progress with my plan, you will start to feel healthier and more confident as your self-esteem increases. You will have more energy and could possibly prevent the onset of more serious medical conditions, such as diabetes, from developing.

Here are some hints and tips to try to keep you motivated:

- **Stand and walk tall.** Keeping your shoulders back, head up and walking tall can help posture. If you look taller, you look slimmer

- **If you have had a good day, or have worked very hard to achieve a substantial weight loss, treat yourself**. You could have a nice relaxing bath, buy your favourite magazine or a new lipstick or treat yourself to a new hairstyle. Maybe you'd like a facial or a manicure? A little pampering will work wonders for your self-esteem

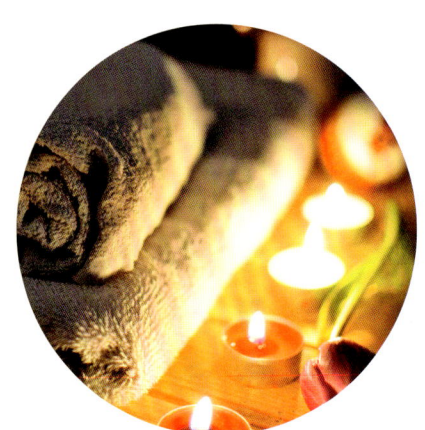

- **Getting good quality sleep is also essential.**
  PCOS sufferers need a good night's sleep. Try going to bed one hour earlier, or if possible, have a nap in the afternoon; you will feel better

- **Avoid eating sugar** it will not help your weight problem or your insulin resistance. Read labels; sometimes sugars are hidden under titles such as 'sorbitol', 'glucose', 'lactose' or 'fructose'. These are all forms of sugar and should be avoided

- **Try, whenever possible, to eat organic fruit, vegetables and good quality protein.** If you cannot afford to do this all the time, treat yourself to organic food just once a week. Think of it as an investment in your health

- **Wash your vegetables and fruit (if not organic) in one part vinegar to twelve parts water.** Rinse in clear cold water to remove the vinegar odour, this can help to reduce the chemicals sprayed on them while they are growing

- **Keep eating your** Nibbles™ — they are the key to your success

- **The diet has been devised to work by increasing your metabolic rate**, so please try to keep exactly to your Healthy Eating and Lifestyle Plan for PCOS and watch the weight come off regularly each week

Top tips for health

Protein

Protein is important for repairing and growing tissue, therefore, you must eat good quality protein. Protein can have a beneficial effect on your insulin levels. When eating meals, it is recommended that you eat a small amount of carbohydrate with your protein (e.g. chicken with vegetables — there are carbohydrates in all vegetables). The absorption of carbohydrates will be slower which means the rise in the level of blood insulin can be minimised.

Good sources of protein are chicken, turkey, oily fish, egg whites and very lean, preferably organic, meats. Animal protein works best because it is full of B vitamins; often depleted in PCOS sufferers due to some of the medicines they take. If you are vegan or vegetarian, susbstitute with your favourite alternatives.

Alcohol

Whilst you are trying to bring the symptoms of PCOS under control, it's a good idea to try to abstain from alcohol. And while a glass of red wine contains bioflavanoids which, together with the alcohol is cardio-protective, exercise can also achieve the same beneficial effect.

Stress

As a PCOS sufferer, you have probably suffered stress because of your symptoms. There is evidence that increased stress levels in PCOS sufferers can make your symptoms worse and cause an increase in insulin resistance. It is therefore important that you try to cut down, or at least try to cope better with the stress in your life. Easier said than done I know, but the tips below should help — they've worked for other sufferers, and they could work for you.

Relieving stress

- Exercise is good for coping with stress
- Meditation or mindfulness are great ways to try and 'get away' from your stress triggers. Make time to practise both. There are lots of videos online that can help you to familiarise yourself with the principles of both
- Alternative therapies such as aromatherapy, acupuncture, NLP and homeopathy can also be useful for managing stress. You may need to experiment to find out which one works best for you. Always consult appropriately qualified professionals before trying alternative medicines or therapies
- Other great stress busters include stretching, deep breathing, positive thinking and chatting with good friends. The most important thing is to start now by finding out whatever suits you. The fact that you have done just that will bring your stress levels down because you are taking steps to improve the quality of your life, by reducing the stress in it

- If the stress becomes too much to take, have a good cry. By crying, you get rid of chemicals in your tears that have been building up during your stressful times
- Herbal teas, camomile or lemon balm all have soothing revitalising properties
- Have a laugh; this is great for stress. Try to think of things in your life that made you really laugh, and re-live or, at least, rethink them. It's a great boost. You could also watch a funny film or comedy series
- People have discovered that stroking the dog, watching a goldfish swimming round a bowl or just relaxing with your eyes closed can help
- Other people find that getting active helps, or going for a long walk on your own to give yourself some space, is good
- Starting a new hobby, or maybe something absorbing such as learning a new language is another idea. Learning something new gives you a focus and stops you from dwelling on the negative aspects that could be causing the stress in your life

Finding the right formula for coping with stress is important to your wellbeing, so start finding what works for you today.

Finally...

When you have PCOS, your system needs regular changes to your diet... so keep varying your food to keep your metabolism working. Each few pounds that you lose will bring about a slight improvement in your health, so it is important that we keep the weight coming off each week.

Smoking

If you smoke, stop now! Smoking produces anti-nutrients and free radicals, which can damage cell membranes in your body and cause other damage.

Smoking is probably the singular, most damaging habit to health. Smoking destroys vitamin C in your body. Burnt, fried or heavily charcoal grilled foods can have a similar effect.

It is important, if you do smoke, that you eat foods rich in vitamin C along with plenty of fresh fruit.

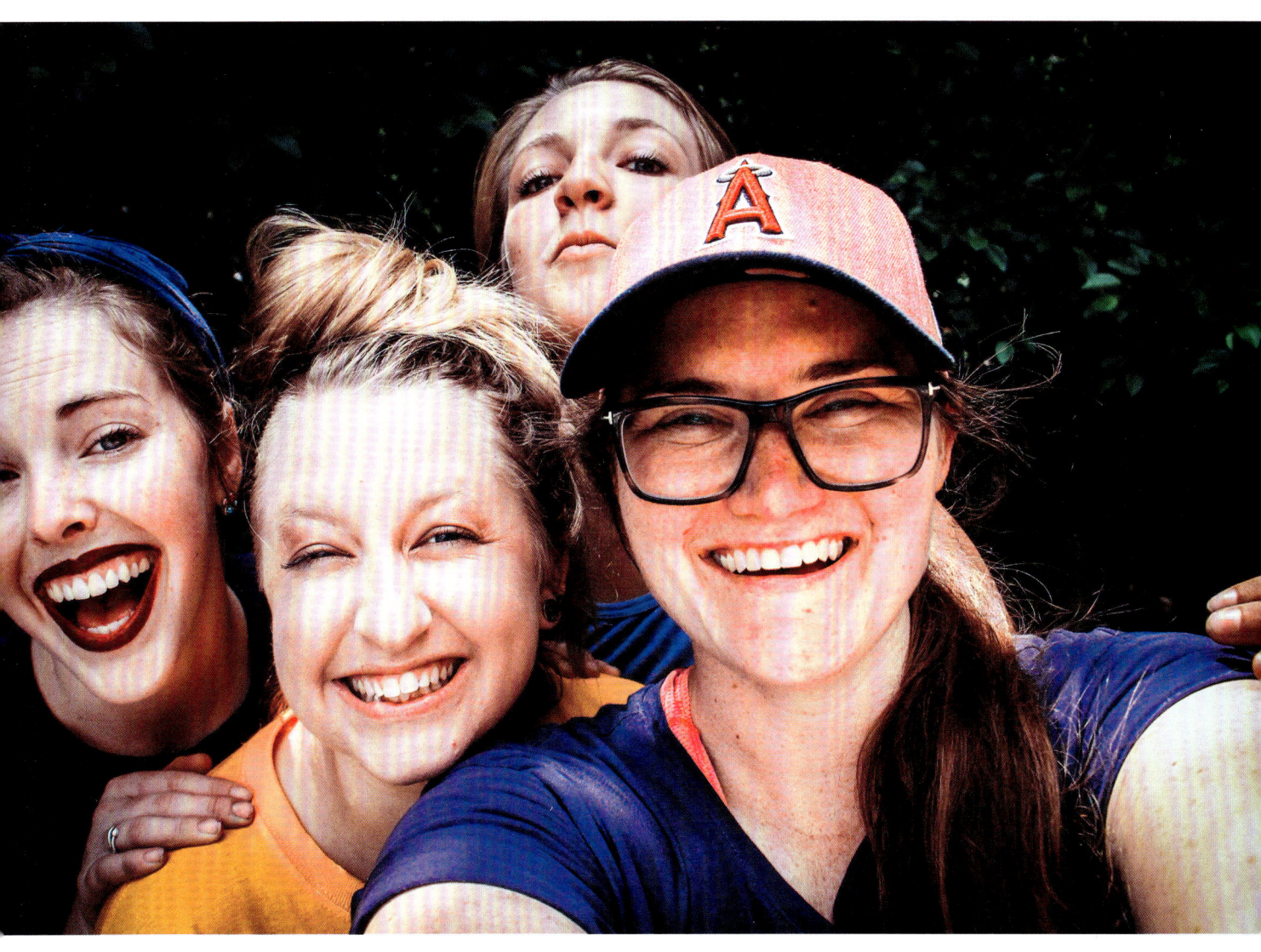

Try to find ways to have fun — it's one of the best ways to relieve stress.

Or feel your stress melting away by watching a funny movie or anything that makes you laugh — there are hundreds of comedies or funny clips to watch online. Netflix, Amazon, YouTube and others have hundreds...it will do you the world of good...who doesn't feel better after a good laugh?

Chapter Seven
The diet

An introduction

The diet essentials

My Healthy Eating and Lifestyle Plan for PCOS is designed to set you on the road to recovery from PCOS by providing you with all the information and tools you need to succeed. Everything has been made as simple as possible for you to understand and follow so that soon you will be 'in control' and your PCOS symptoms can at last become manageable.

> **Please note:**
>
> You must eat to lose weight
>
> You will be eating more than usual
>
> You will NEVER be hungry on this diet (unless you have an extraordinarily large appetite)

First things first:

- If you have a tendency to binge — MAKE SURE you read the chapter on Bingeing and follow my Binge Recovery Guide (page 29) to ditch bingeing forever!

- Read 'Before you start' on page 69 — it will set you up for success!

- Take a look at which foods you are allowed on the diet (page 98)

- Look at the meal plans to decide which foods to buy in

- Use your shopping list on page 86 for your essentials

In this chapter

Your shopping list

Choose organic

Essential: Nibbles™ and Burns™

Frequently Asked Questions on Nibbles™ and Burns™

Your shopping list

Here is a list of items you will need to start your diet.

Please try to buy organic produce.

- ☑ **Fresh fruit** — pears and kiwis are good choices
- ☑ **Breakfast cereals** — select from cereal options on page 103
- ☑ **Protein foods** — see page 100
- ☑ **Fresh vegetables** — select from vegetables list on page 99
- ☑ **Salad** — Choose tomatoes, lettuce, cucumber, cress, spring onions
- ☑ **Peppers** — Red, Orange, and Yellow for your Nibbles™
- ☑ **Crispbreads** — Rye, corn crispbreads or rice cakes
- ☑ **Lemon or lime** — Preferably unwaxed
- ☑ **Milk** — Full fat dairy or unsweetened plant milk (organic)
- ☑ **Cottage cheese** — Includes varieties
- ☑ **Organic stock cubes**
- ☑ **Drinks** — Still water, decaffeinated tea or coffee, herbal teas, fruit teas, low calorie cordials and fresh fruit juices
- ☑ **Organic yoghurt**
- ☑ **Vinegar**
- ☑ **Herbs and spices**
- ☑ **Berries**
- ☑ **Seeds**
- ☑ **Butter**
- ☑ **Olive oil**
- ☑ **Exfoliating mitts**

Happy shopping!

Choose organic

Because PCOS sufferers have a chemical imbalance, foods that have been sprayed with chemicals or contain artificial hormones and steroids can only make their chemical imbalances worse.

The benefits of eating organic food for PCOS should not therefore be underestimated. That's why choosing to eat organic is one of the main principles of my Healthy Eating and Lifestyle Plan for PCOS.

According to the UK Soil Association, organic food is better for your health.

Organically-grown foods come from farms that use farming techniques that are sustainable and support the environment. The result is good quality soil that is mineral rich for growing crops. Organically-grown vegetables are more nutrient dense and are free from chemical toxins.

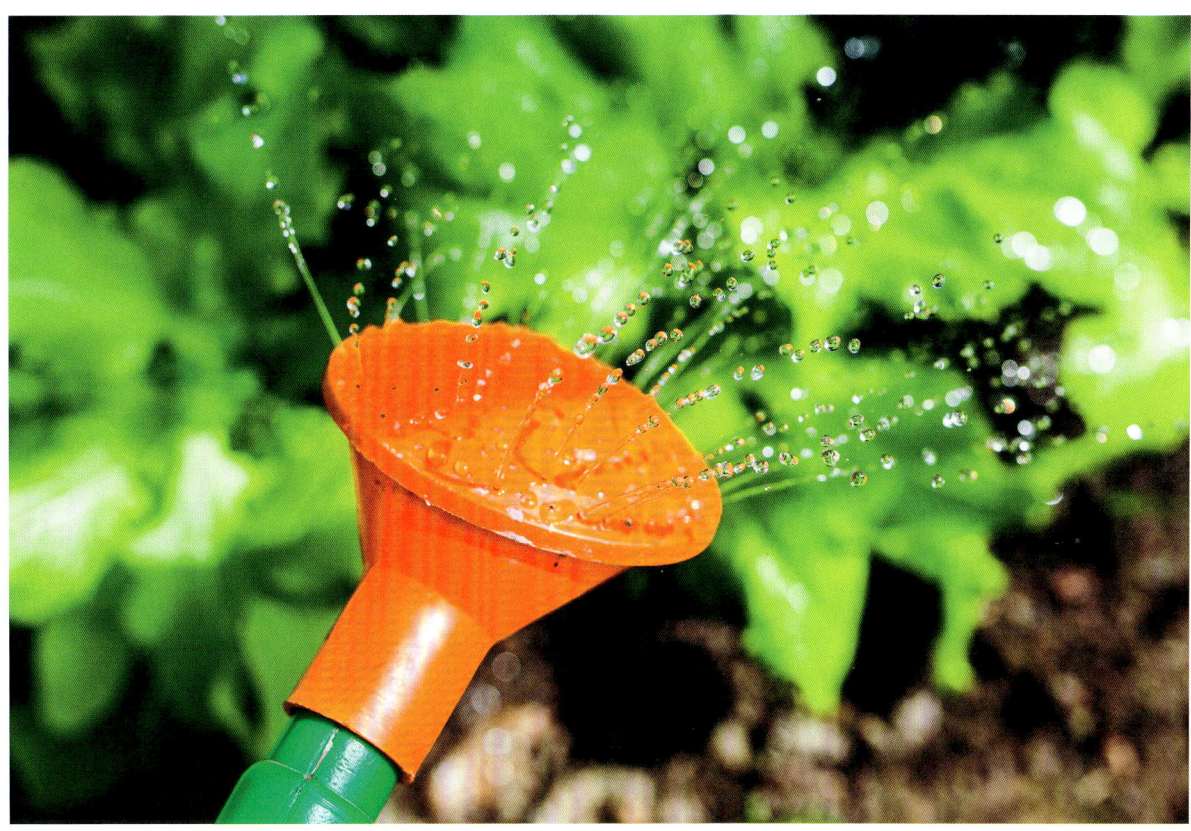

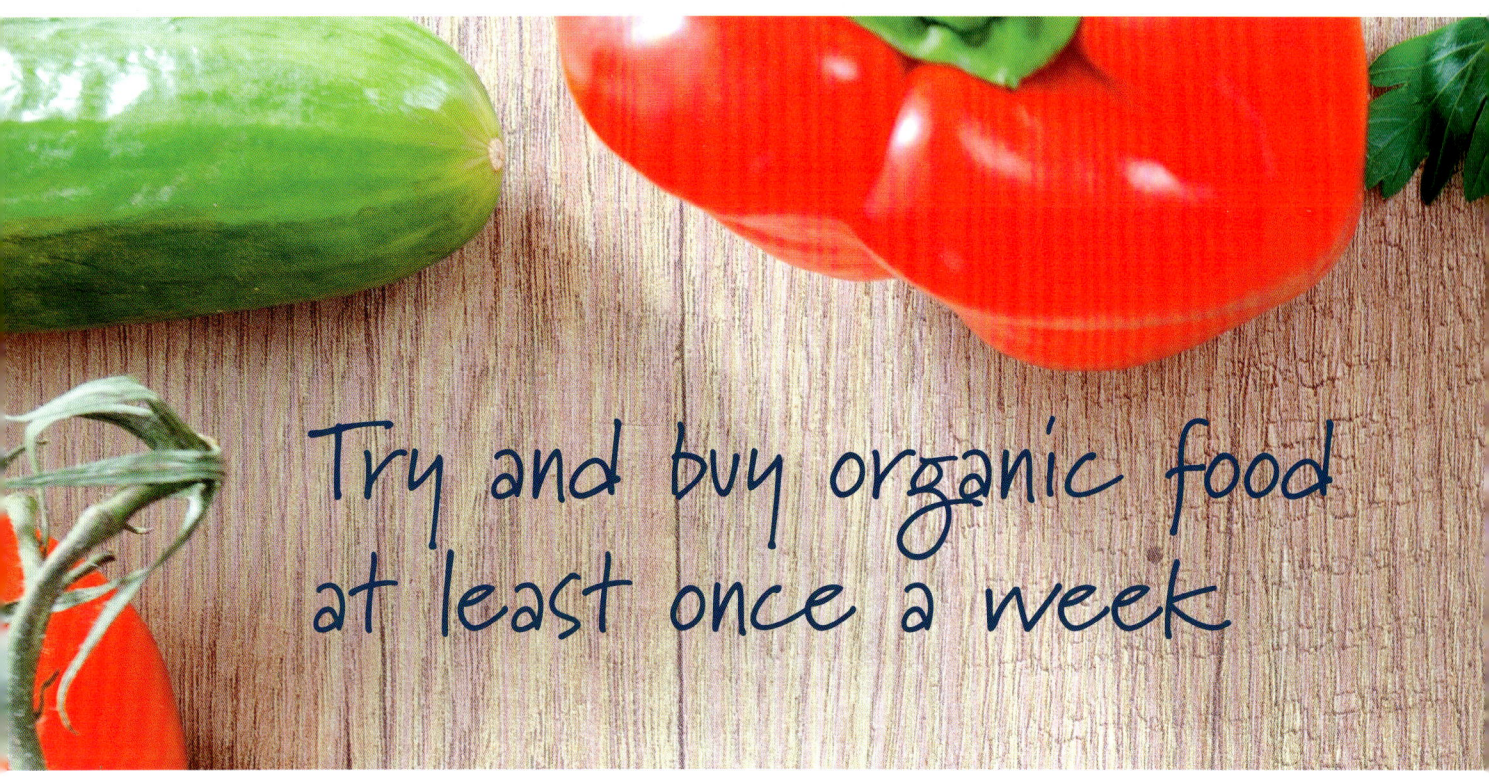

Try and buy organic food at least once a week

Animals that are not organically reared are only as good as the grass and animal feed they eat. Intensively-farmed animals do not get to use their muscles normally, as they are often kept in very cramped, overcrowded enclosures. Often fed steroids, their meat is inevitably fattier.

Organically-reared livestock, allowed to roam and find food naturally, have considerably leaner meat than intensively farmed animals.

The heavier an animal is, the better the price in the marketplace. The fat that we consume from animals is mainly saturated fat. According to advice from the UK's National Health Service and Cancer Research UK, saturated fat is one of the types of fat we should be trying to reduce within our diets, so eating organically-grown meats reduces your saturated fat intake and avoids exposure to other non-food chemicals.

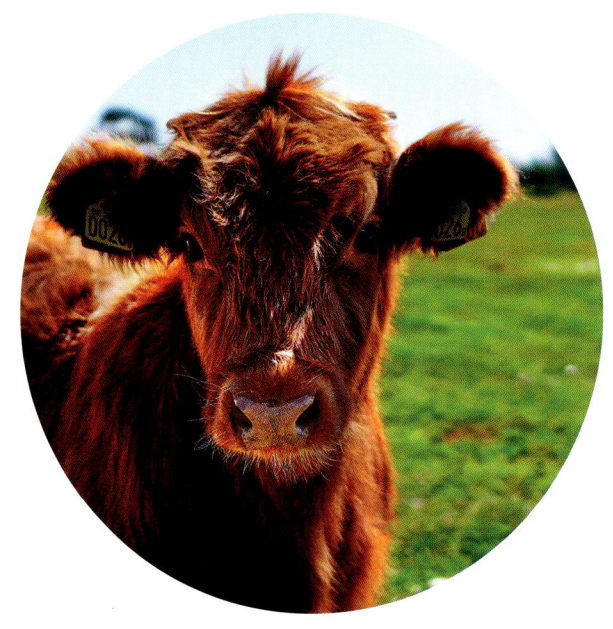

Organic foods are not only more nutrient dense, those nutrients are of a better quality. Most UK supermarkets sell a lot of organic produce.

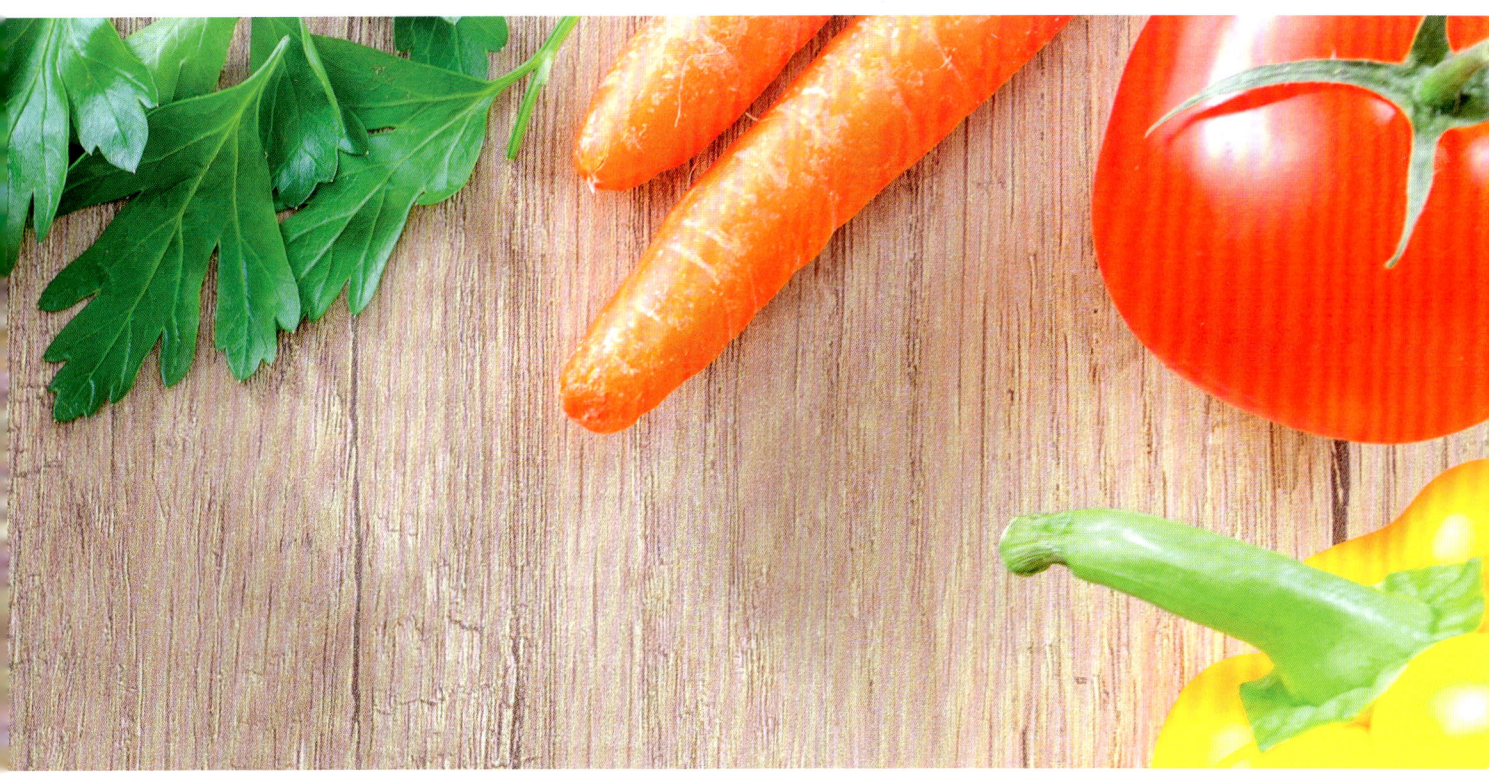

Get into the habit of looking at organic food as an investment in your health. If you cannot afford or cannot find organic fruit and vegetables, make sure you wash all fruit and vegetables really well. Do this in a mixture of twelve parts water to a capful of organic cider vinegar. When you have washed, rinse again, to remove the odour of the vinegar on your food.

You can also buy specialist products, designed to help get rid of some of the pesticides and germs. It is worth peeling vegetables such as carrots, which have been found to contain a large amount of chemical residue, in their outer skin.

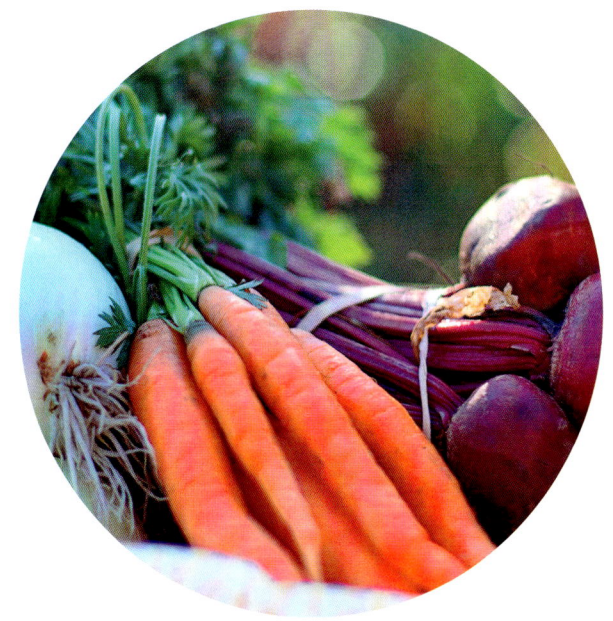

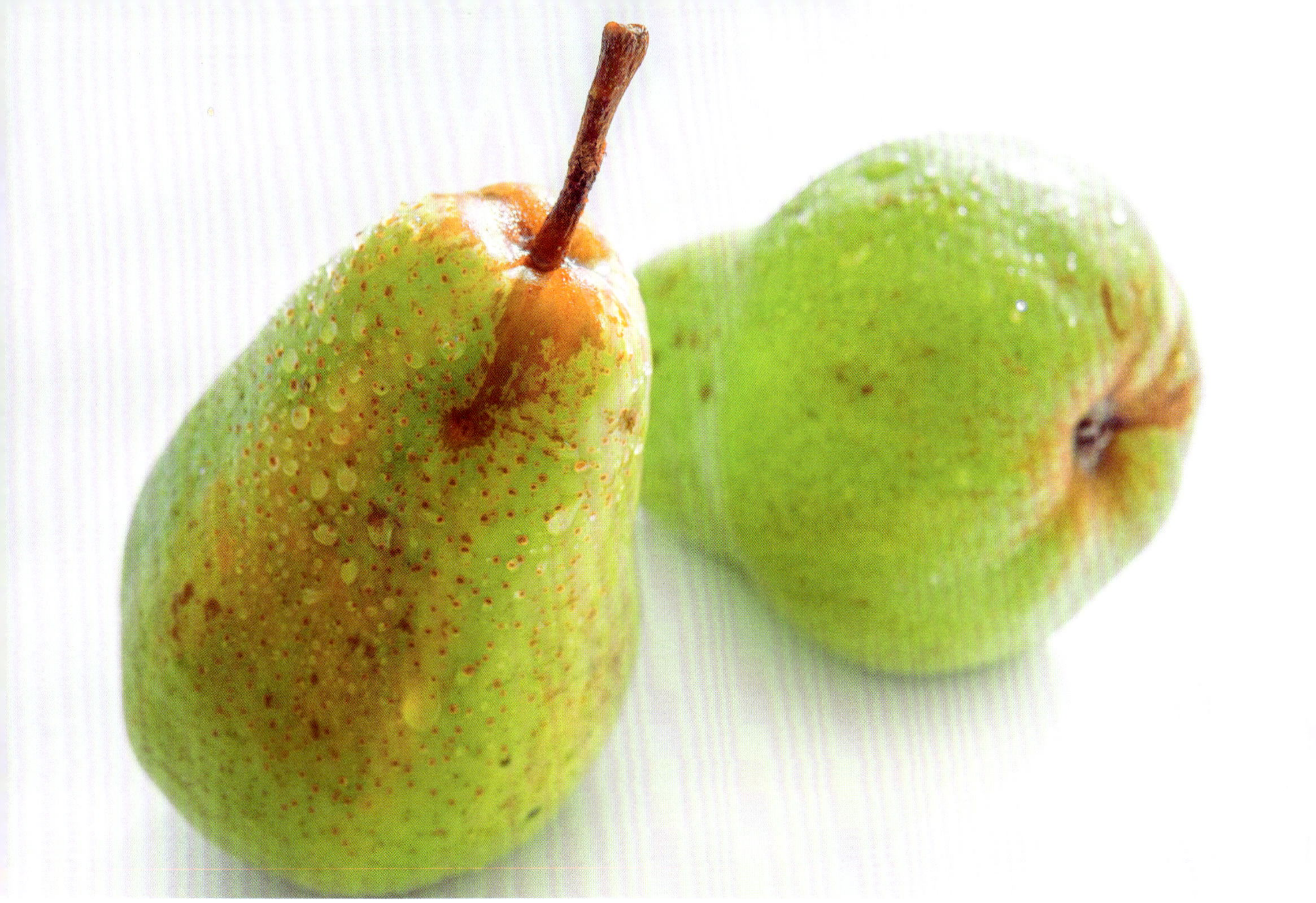

Kiwi and pear are the best fruits to eat — they are **full** of essential vitamins

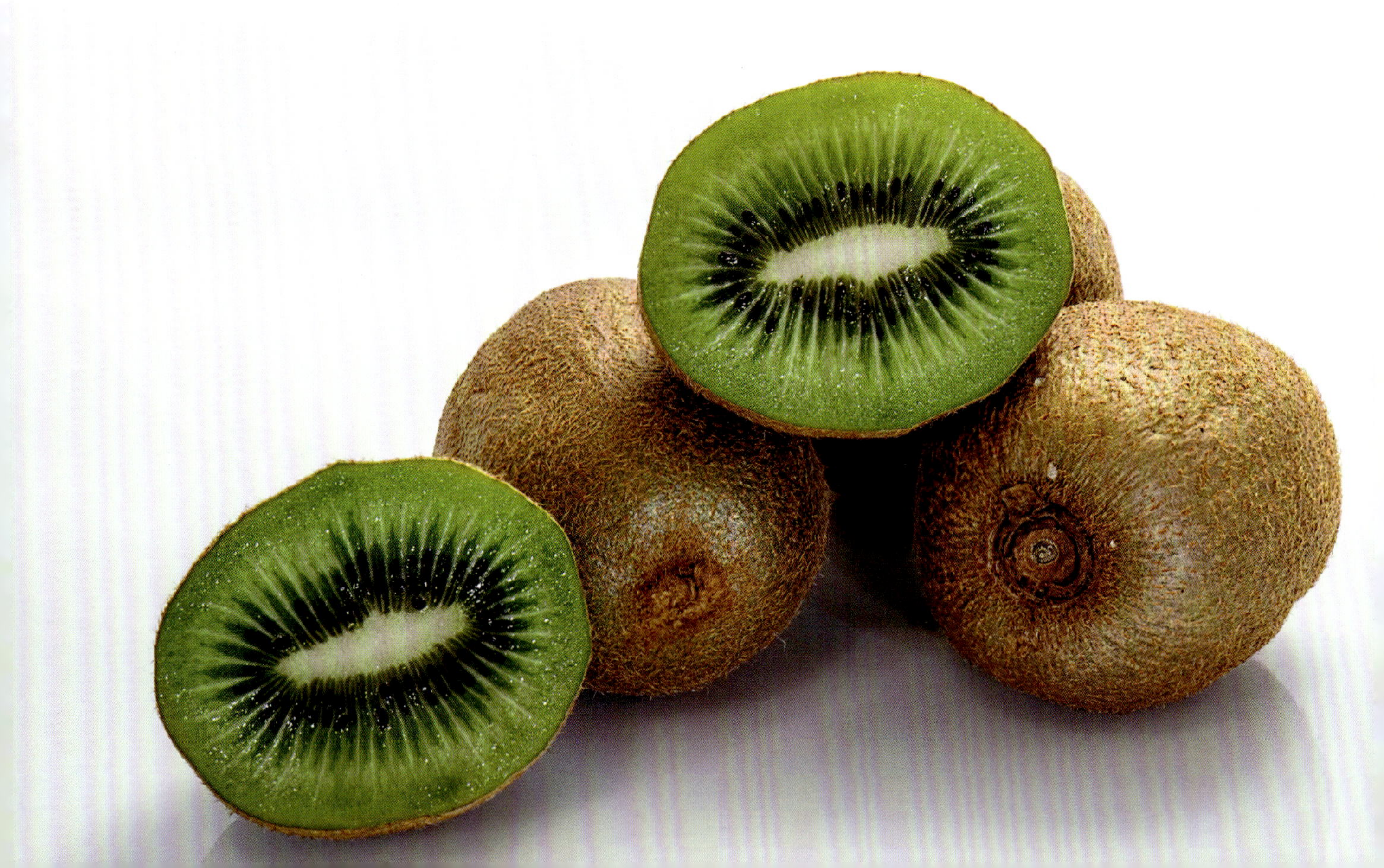

Essential: Your Nibbles™ and Burns™

Essential to my Healthy Eating and Lifestyle Plan for PCOS are what I call Nibbles™ and Burns™. These are very small pieces of vegetable (Nibbles™) and very small pieces of protein (Burns™). Eating a Nibble™ or a Burn™ every 15 minutes can boost your metabolism as well as bombard your body with essential vitamins which can help you lose weight. Losing weight can improve insulin levels and stop you feeling hungry or craving food.

The importance of your Nibbles™ and Burns™ cannot be stressed enough — they are **essential** to your weight loss. Make sure you include them in your daily regime. They can help 'fire up' your metabolism. Remember as a PCOS sufferer you have a very sluggish metabolic rate which means your metabolism can be slow and you will be unable to burn off much of what you eat.

Nibbles™

Here is a list of the best vegetable Nibbles™ to choose from (preferably organic).

- Peppers (choose from red, orange and yellow — green peppers can be bitter tasting)
- Cucumber
- Carrots (raw)
- Celery (raw)
- White cabbage (raw)
- Cauliflower (raw)
- Courgette (raw)
- Mange tout (raw)
- Green beans (raw)
- Broccoli (raw)
- Blueberries

Every  **15 mins**

> **Important:** Your Nibbles™ should be tiny. The smaller the Nibble™, the better the weight loss — imagine a small postage stamp folded into four — that is the size to aim for.

> **Important:** Set an alarm on your phone so you remember to eat your Nibbles™ or Burns™ every 15 minutes. Prepare them first thing in the morning — so they are ready as soon as you've had breakfast — they are so important to your success!

Introducing the 'ROY' technique

For best results on the diet, from Day 1, use the ROY (Red, Orange and Yellow peppers) technique as follows:

Day 1: Nibble™ on **Red** peppers

Day 2: Nibble™ on **Orange** peppers

Day 3: Nibble™ on **Yellow** peppers

Days 4-7: Alternate your Nibbles™ with a mixture of all three

If you don't like peppers, choose something else from your vegetable Nibbles™ list on page 91.

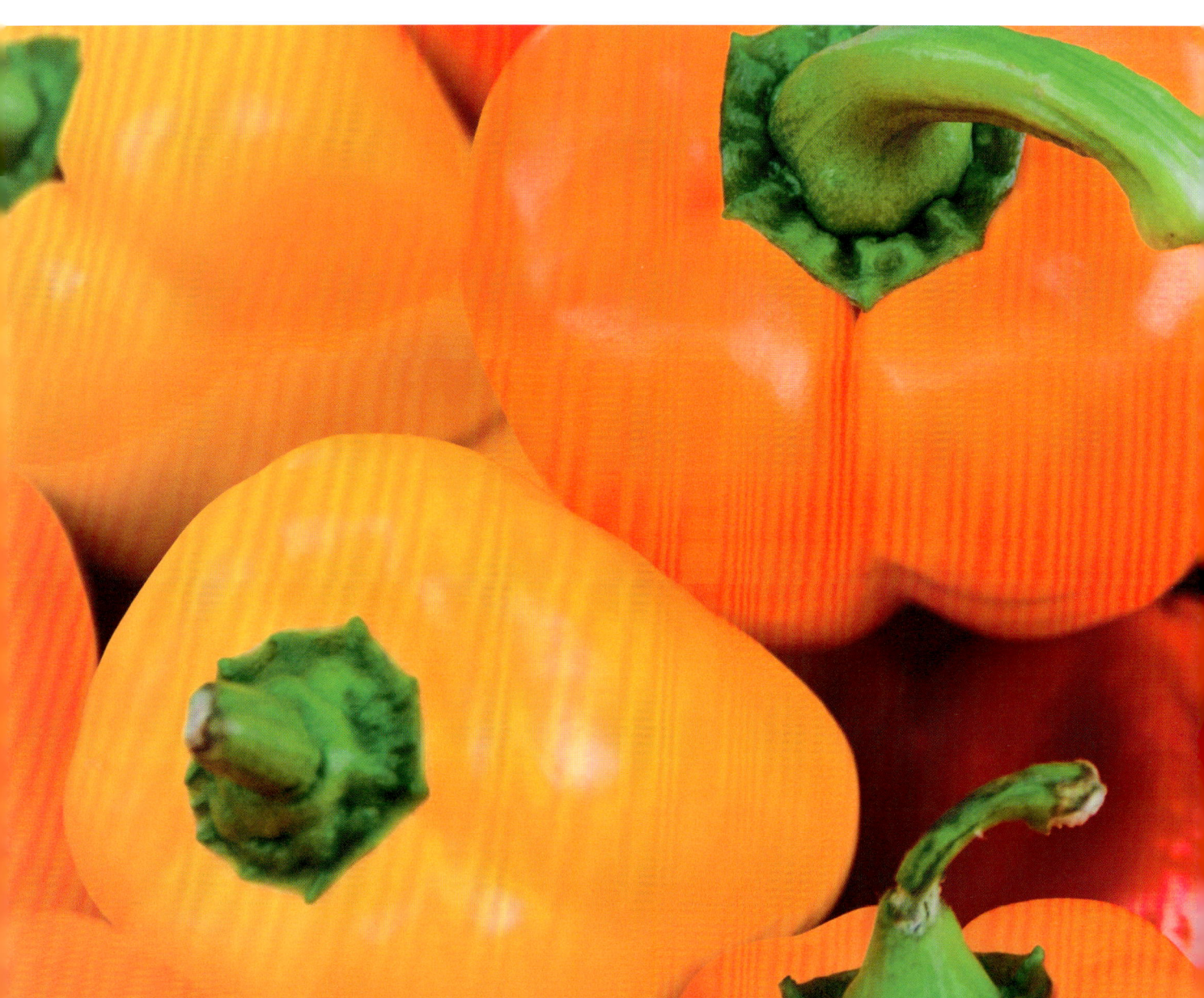

Burns™

Start your Burns™ after a weight loss of 4.5-6 kg/10-14 lbs (usually two to three weeks into the plan).

Burns™ are proteins such as:

- Almond flakes (as long as you don't have a nut allergy)
- Cottage cheese
- Fish
- Chicken or any poultry
- Egg
- Any lean cooked meat (unprocessed)
- Liver
- Any organic meat e.g. steak, pork, lamb or beef

Every

15 mins

Animal protein contains B vitamins. Some PCOS sufferers, especially those taking medication, can find that their body has insufficient levels of B vitamins. Protein Burns™ can help speed up the metabolism. Animal protein Burns™ can replenish your body with these essential vitamins needed for good health.

'This PCOS healthy eating plan had helped my elder sister so when I was diagnosed with PCOS, I decided to give it a try. Four stone lighter in six months, after eating healthy food. I was never hungry.'

Sarah, Liverpool

Frequently asked questions on Nibbles™ and Burns™

What are Nibbles™ and Burns™?

Nibbles™ are little pieces of vegetable like peppers, carrots or cucumber (see page 91 for a list). Burns™ are little pieces of protein, like almond flakes, chicken (any poultry), fish, egg and cottage cheese.

How big should a Nibble™ or Burn™ be?

No bigger than a small postage stamp, folded into four, the tinier the better.

Why do I have to eat a Nibble™ or a Burn™ every 15 minutes?

15 minutes after you've eaten your Nibble™ or Burn™, your metabolism will have slowed again. That is why it is extremely important to keep eating a Nibble™ or a Burn™ every 15 minutes – it can help keep your metabolism burning **all day long** and can help to level your blood sugars while giving you energy as you bombard your body with essential vitamins.

What happens if I cannot manage to eat a Nibble™ or a Burn™ every 15 minutes?

This can slow your weight loss down. Eating a Nibble™ or Burn™ every 15 minutes can make a really big difference to your weight loss, but doing just a few during the course of the day/evening is better than none at all.

Does it matter which one you start with?

Yes. You **must** start with vegetable Nibbles™ — see the ROY technique on page 92.

Why do I need to start with vegetable Nibbles™?

If you carry any excess weight (not all PCOS sufferers are overweight); some of it will be fluid or water retention. If you suffer with fluid retention, vegetable Nibbles™ are best because vegetables can help your body to expel excess fluid.

When can I start with my protein Burns™?

When you have started to lose weight, say 4.5-6 kg/10-14 lbs, you then need to change to your Burns™ to continue your weight loss.

As a PCOS sufferer, you may be on medication due to hormone imbalances and insulin resistance. Some medicines can affect your absorption of certain vitamins, especially some of the B vitamins – animal protein is full of these vitamins. Your Burns™, when taken in tiny amounts, every 15 minutes will bombard your body with vitamins which are so essential for your health.

Chapter Eight
The 'new you' begins

The 'new you' begins here with your complete PCOS diet for immediate weight loss

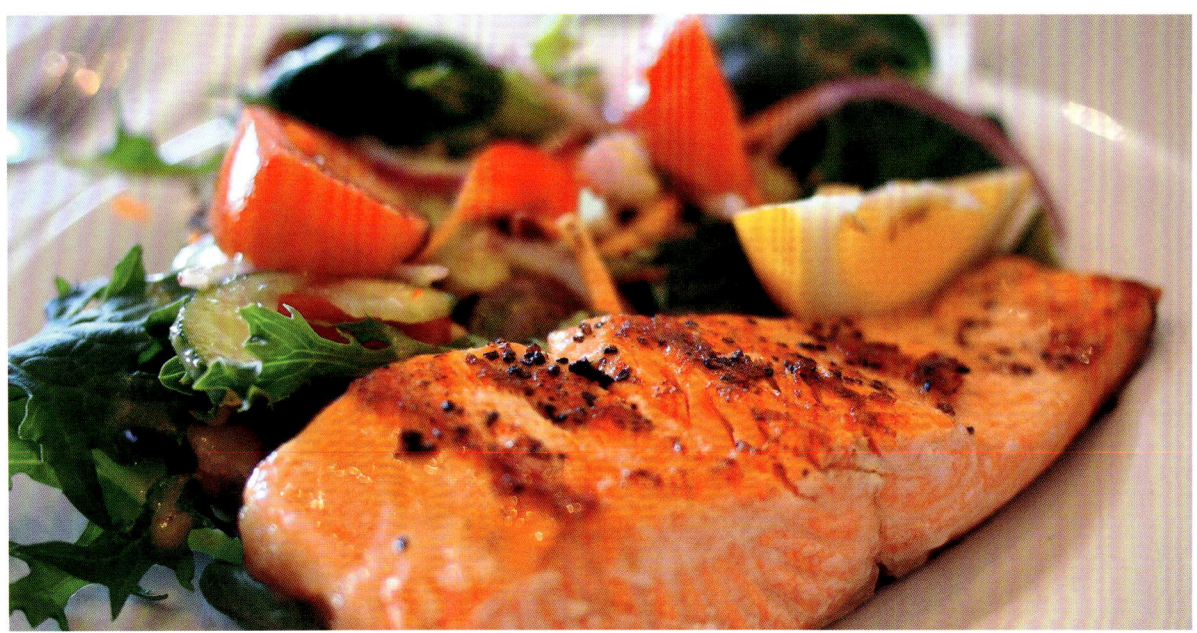

After following the diet for a few weeks you will begin to alter your relationship with food and develop lifestyle habits that can help you control your PCOS symptoms. You will also be bombarding your body with nutrients helping it to do its job of cleansing and boosting your overall health.

In this chapter

What and how much to eat (includes meal plans)

Breakfast

Mid-morning snack

Lunch

Mid-afternoon snack

Evening meal

Evening snack/supper

Important things to note...

- Follow the diet **exactly**
- Do **not** miss any meals (doing so can **SLOW** your metabolism down)
- No alcohol but don't despair — it's just temporary. You will be able to drink a glass of wine every day once you start to lose weight. The weight loss will happen in the first week if you follow the guidance exactly
- Do **not** eat any bread (PCOS sufferers are sensitive to wheat. flour and yeast. If you can't live without any one of these, you can start eating them again in moderation, once you have made good progress with your weight loss. You can eat rye crispbreads and rice cakes on the diet — but no wheat)
- Avoid pasta and rice. Your metabolic rate may be very slow which could mean you are unable to burn off these carbohydrates; especially if eaten in the evening
- Do not eat potatoes in the evening — you won't have time to burn off the carbohydrate before bedtime
- Do not eat mashed potatoes, chips or fries. Eat jacket potatoes instead, with the skin for added fibre, but no later than lunchtime
- Lunch and evening meals can be swapped if more convenient
- Vary your meals by choosing a different breakfast, lunch and evening meal every day. It will help with your weight loss because it kickstarts the system and can speed up your metabolic rate
- For maximum results stick to exact amounts for all carbohydrates in the diet
- Add a **paper thin** slice of lemon or lime to hot water and leave for four hours or overnight before drinking each morning before food. **If you suffer from arthritis please do not drink lemon or lime water**
- Drink decaffeinated coffee, or green or herbal teas. Any low calorie drinks diluted with plenty of water, also still water. If eating any cold food it is preferable to have a hot drink beforehand
- Make homemade, organic, vegetable soup that you can have anytime you feel hungry (see soup recipes on page 147)
- Do not thicken sauces or gravies with flour or thickening products as this will slow down your progress
- Eat 7.5 cm/3 inches of cucumber that has been marinated in vinegar (the equivalent in pickled gherkins). It will help you shed unwanted fluid you could be holding on to. Use peppers or celery if you don't like cucumber. If you have arthritic problems, omit the vinegar and eat 10 cm/4 inches of cucumber instead
- Eat some extra protein if you feel hungry such as some chicken or a couple of tablespoons of cottage cheese, or a bowl of homemade soup without thickener, starch or potatoes
- Avoid fizzy or carbonated drinks. These can increase hunger and affect hormone imbalances

What and how much to eat (includes meal plans)

Your daily allowances

- 284 ml/½ pint of organic milk
- 14 g/½ oz butter (grass fed is best) or 1 tablespoon of mayonnaise/olive oil/cream/2 tablespoons plain organic yoghurt
- 3 fresh fruits (pears and kiwis are good choices)
- 2-3 portions of vegetables (see allowed vegetables list on page 99)
- 10 blueberries/other berries
- ¼ teaspoon of seeds (sunflower, linseed, flax, sesame, pumpkin or mixed)

Tips:

- Stir fry food with fine spray oils
- Avoid citrus fruits like oranges and grapefruit if you suffer with acid in your digestive tract or if you have arthritis
- You are allowed one baked potato at lunch time (do not eat any starch later than lunch time because you will be unlikely to burn it off before bedtime)
- If you have more than 19 kg/42 lbs to lose, it is better to avoid eating any cooked root vegetables (you can however, eat raw carrots as Nibbles™)
- Raw vegetables from your allowed vegetable foods list (see page 99) are a good source of fibre which helps to cleanse your system
- No more than three pieces of fresh fruit to be eaten daily, (no bananas or cherries)

Vegetables allowed on the diet

- Asparagus
- Aubergine
- Beansprouts
- Broccoli
- Cabbage
- Cauliflower
- Chinese leaves
- Courgettes
- Cucumber
- Green Beans
- Lettuce
- Mange tout
- Mushrooms
- Mustard cress
- Peppers (red/orange/green/yellow)
- Spinach
- Sprouts
- Vegetable marrow
- Watercress

'When my weight ballooned to over 20 stone, and my PCOS symptoms were stopping me functioning like a normal woman, I stopped going out. My social life was non-existent. Norah helped me not only to lose weight and reduce the PCOS unpleasant symptoms, but she taught me how to keep control of my new figure without constantly being pre-occupied with food. I lost seven stone in 12 months and won a dancing competition.'

Angela, Manchester UK

Proteins allowed on the diet

Meat
- Lamb
- Beef
- Pork
- Ham and other unprocessed cooked meats

Poultry (remove skin)
- Chicken
- Turkey
- Duck
- Goose

Other
- Rabbit
- Offal
- Liver
- Kidney

- Fish (fresh and tinned) — All fish; but no batter, breadcrumbs or sauces and drain oil from tinned fish
- Cottage cheese — all varieties
- 28 g/1 oz hard cheese daily. Omit all hard cheese if on any medication, as it can slow your metabolism down and consequently your weight loss
- All light cheeses, for example soft spreading cheeses
- Eggs, boiled, poached or scrambled

Tip: Be sure to read the label to avoid any processed meats.

Due to medications, PCOS sufferers often have a shortage of B vitamins; animal protein is a great source of B vitamins and is therefore highly recommended on this diet.

NOTE:
You do not have to be strict about weighing out your protein or your vegetables, but as a guideline, your protein and vegetable allowance should be approximately 113 g/4 oz per portion, when cooked.

Tips: Remove fat from meats to improve your weight loss. Remove the skin from chicken.

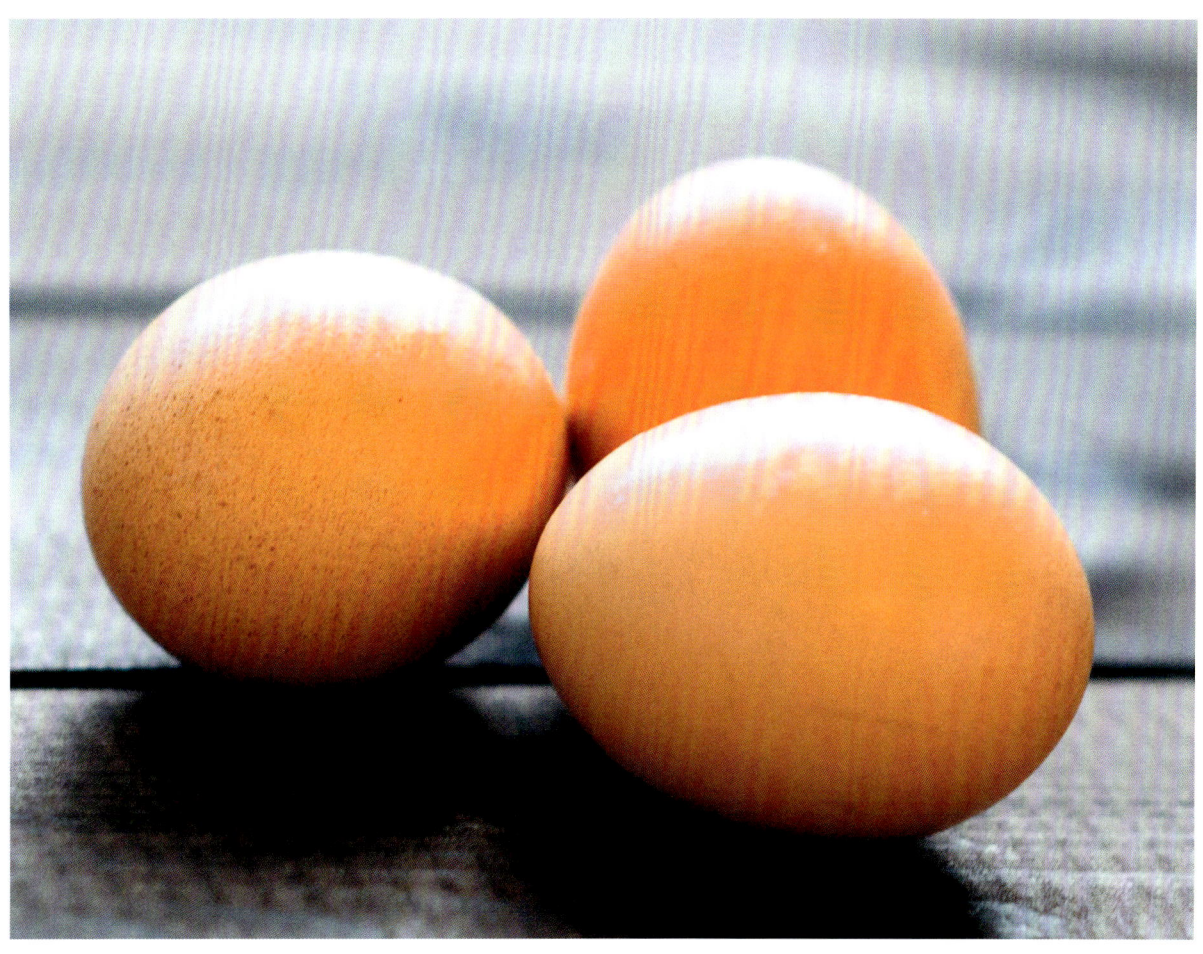

Tip: Hard boil some eggs. They are a good source of protein. If you suffer with high cholesterol only have three egg yolks a week but as many egg whites as you desire.

Egg whites make excellent Burns™.

Breakfast

Before Breakfast

Ensure you drink your glass of boiled, cooled, water which has been poured over a **paper thin** slice of lemon or lime, and left overnight to infuse.

Do your gentle exercises morning and evening as set out in Getting Active (see page 108).

Drink decaffeinated coffee or tea with your breakfast with a small amount of milk, but no sugar. If you prefer you could substitute the tea or coffee for fresh water but no fizzy or carbonated drinks.

Immediately after breakfast, start your Nibbles™ and eat one every 15 minutes. If you cannot nibble because of circumstances, then nibble at night, weekend, or whenever you can.

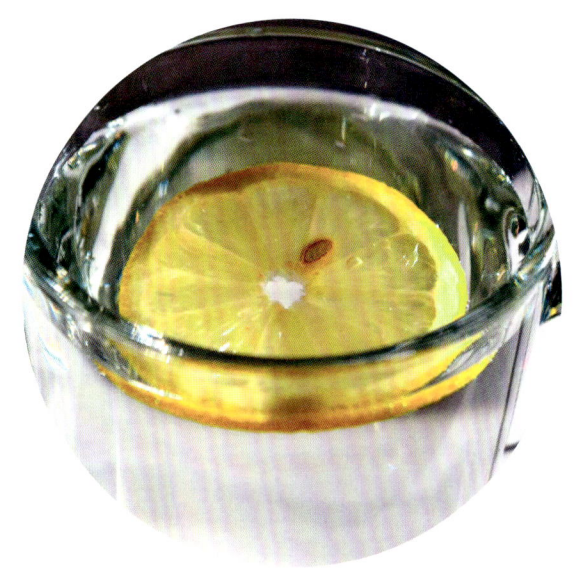

Add a **paper thin** slice of lemon or lime to a glass of hot water and leave for four hours, preferably overnight. Leave it on your bedside cabinet and drink first thing in the morning. Keep topping it up throughout the day to stay hydrated.

DISCLAIMER

Following the advice to drink lemon or lime water as recommended, is at your own discretion. It is understood that by following the advice to drink lemon or lime water, you accept this disclaimer.

Tips:

- Do not miss breakfast, it's important for your weight loss
- For a quicker weight loss choose a different breakfast daily
- Use hot milk on your cereal
- Add 10 blueberries and ¼ teaspoon of seeds to all breakfast cereals

Your breakfast choices

NB: Please add 10 berries and a ¼ teaspoon of seeds to your breakfast cereals OR include them in a salad later in the day.

Breakfast 1	Mix together 3 heaped tablespoons of plain Special K with 3 heaped tablespoons of bran flakes. Pour over a small amount of preferably, hot milk. Add sweetener if required. If you don't like Special K or Bran Flakes just have 6 tablespoons of any plain, sugar free cereal.
Breakfast 2	1 Weetabix or Shredded Wheat, with milk, and sweetener if required.
Breakfast 3	28 g/1 oz of any plain breakfast cereal, without sugar, such as All Bran, Cornflakes, Rice Krispies or sugar reduced Muesli — you can mix cereals together if preferred.
Breakfast 4	3 heaped tablespoons of plain porridge, (uncooked).
Breakfast 5	2 crispbreads OR 2 rice cakes. Top with cottage cheese or any protein topping. PLUS 1 small pear or 113 g/4 oz of another fresh fruit (avoid bananas and cherries).
Breakfast 6	2 fresh fruit, such as, oranges, or grapefruit, chopped and warmed (you can add a tablespoon of plain yoghurt if desired). PLUS 10 berries and ¼ teaspoon of any seeds. AND 1 crispbread. If you suffer from arthritis, citrus fruit should be avoided because of the acid — eat apples, pears, peaches, or kiwi fruit instead.
Breakfast 7	1 scrambled, boiled or poached egg. 1 rasher of bacon. 1 high-meat content sausage. 1 tomato. A small portion of mushrooms.

Please select a different breakfast every day to vary your diet and boost your metabolism.

Immediately after breakfast start your Nibbles™ and eat one every 15 minutes where possible. Follow the ROY technique on page 92 and start Day 1 on my plan with a Red pepper, Day 2 an Orange pepper, Day 3 a Yellow pepper and then mix them all together and choose from any one of them, for the rest of the week.

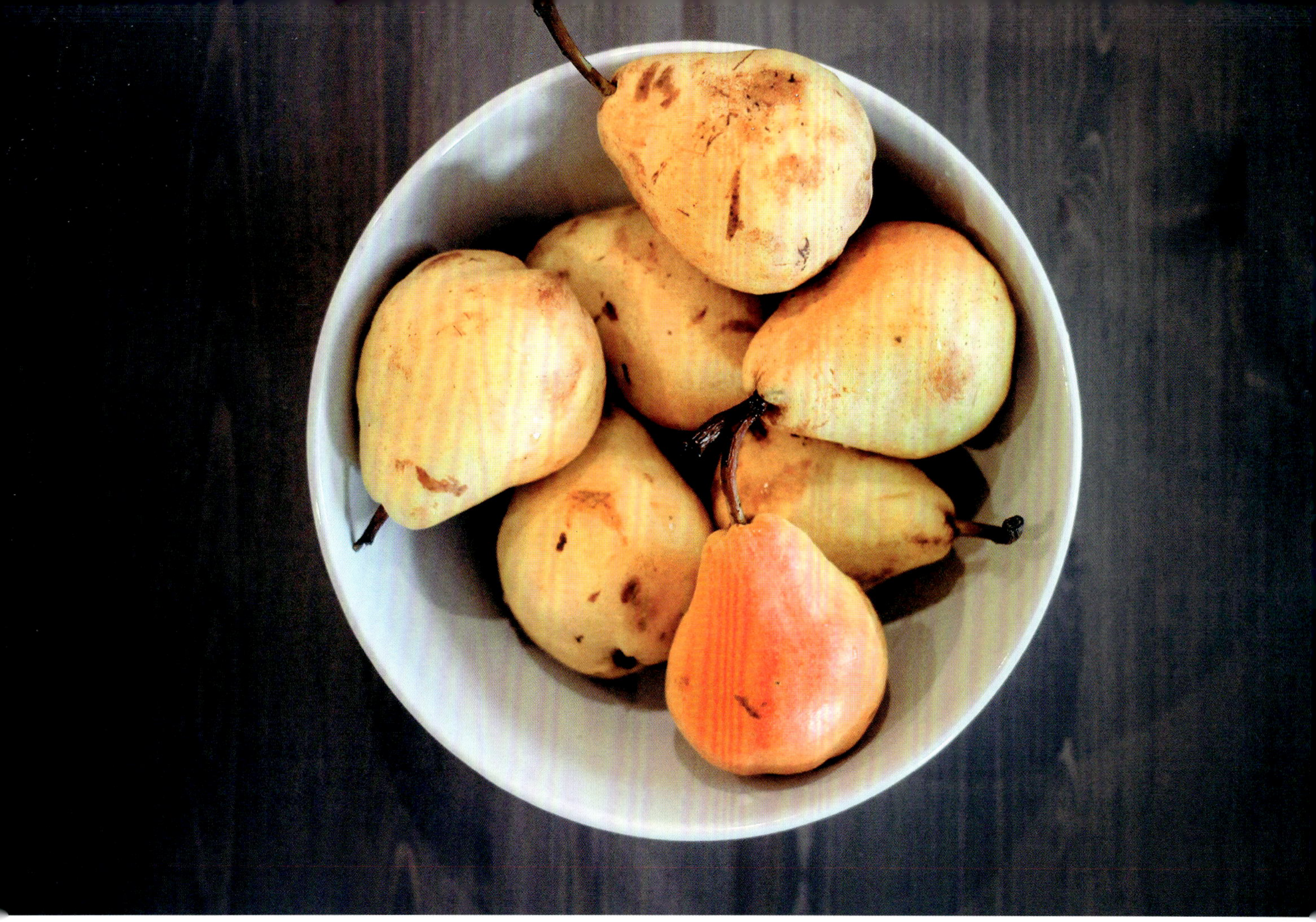

Mid-morning snack

Do not miss your mid-morning snack. Preferably you should eat a piece of fresh, organic fruit. A pear or kiwi would be a good choice. After your fruit:

- Have a permitted drink
- Continue with your Nibbles™

> **Tips:**
> - Your Nibbles™ can help to cleanse your body and help you lose excess fluid
> - After three days on ROY (Red, Orange and Yellow) pepper Nibbles™; prepare a mixture of all three colours to choose from randomly. Varying your Nibbles™ can stimulate your metabolism and help you lose excess weight faster

Lunch

Select a lunch from the list below. Try to vary your meals. If the weather is cold, start with homemade soup in place of a piece of fruit from your daily fruit allowance.

Lunch 1	3 crispbreads or rice cakes, with a choice of the following toppings:
	- Tuna, salmon, or any fish, tinned or fresh (drain oil)
	- Cottage cheese (any variety)
	- Any unprocessed, cooked meat
	- Any low calorie spread, such as cream cheese
	- Any protein topping from the allowed proteins' list on page 100
	- Include a small salad made of:
	  - Lettuce
	  - Cucumber
	  - 1 Tomato, watercress, spring onions

Lunch 2	1 sandwich made with 2 small slices of yeast-free bread. This could be rye bread topped with any of the protein fillings mentioned in Lunch 1, including the salad.
Lunch 3	A 227g/8 oz (when raw), jacket potato, (when cooked the potato will be approximately 142 g/5 oz) with a protein topping, such as cottage cheese or tuna. You could select any protein topping from your list on page 100, plus the salad from Lunch 1, above.
Lunch 4	113g/4 oz of good quality protein (see allowed proteins' list on page 100), and the salad from Lunch 1 or vegetables, of your choice, (see allowed vegetables list on page 99).
Lunch 5	1 piece of toast, yeast free bread, such as rye, with a protein topping, such as tuna or egg, plus the salad from Lunch 1, above.

Tip: Make a soup using the water you cooked your vegetables in. Add some chicken to make a Burns™ soup. It will be cheaper and much healthier than packet soups (see soup recipes page 147).

IMPORTANT: If eating a cold meal, have a hot drink or hot soup first to improve weight loss.

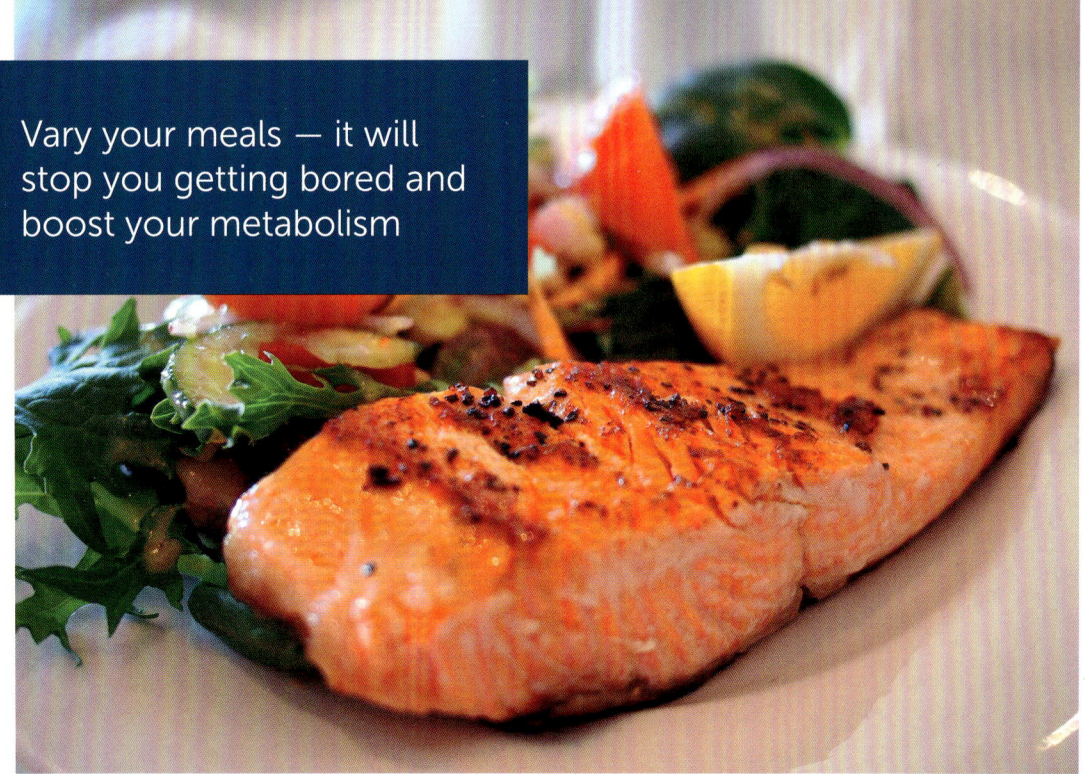

Vary your meals — it will stop you getting bored and boost your metabolism

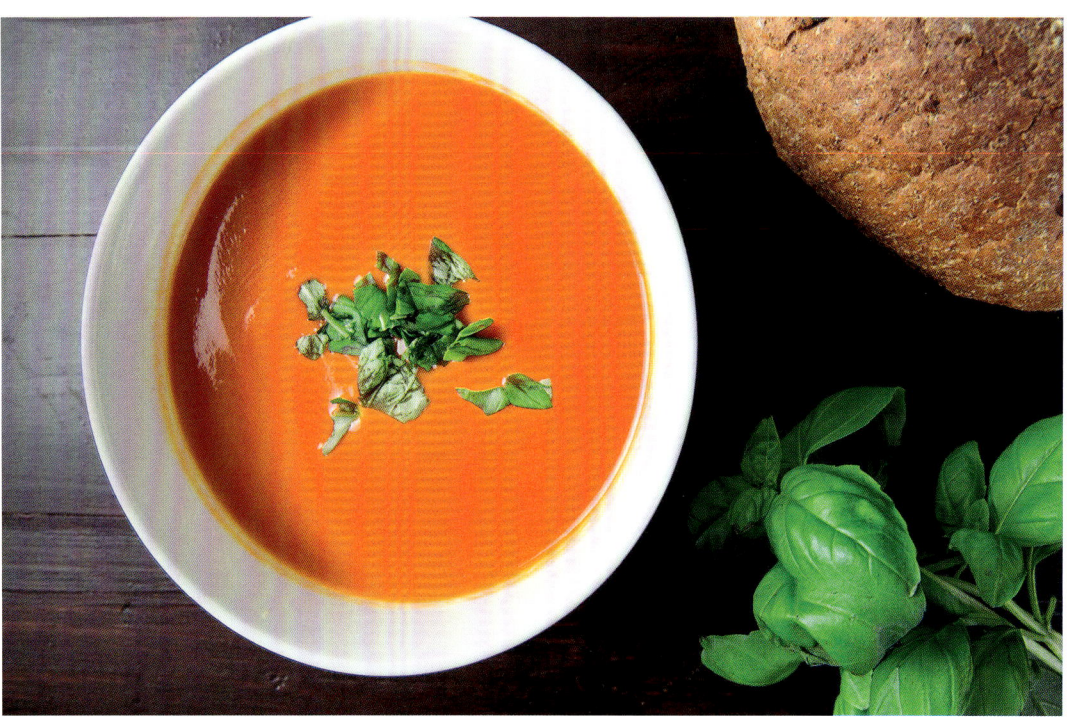

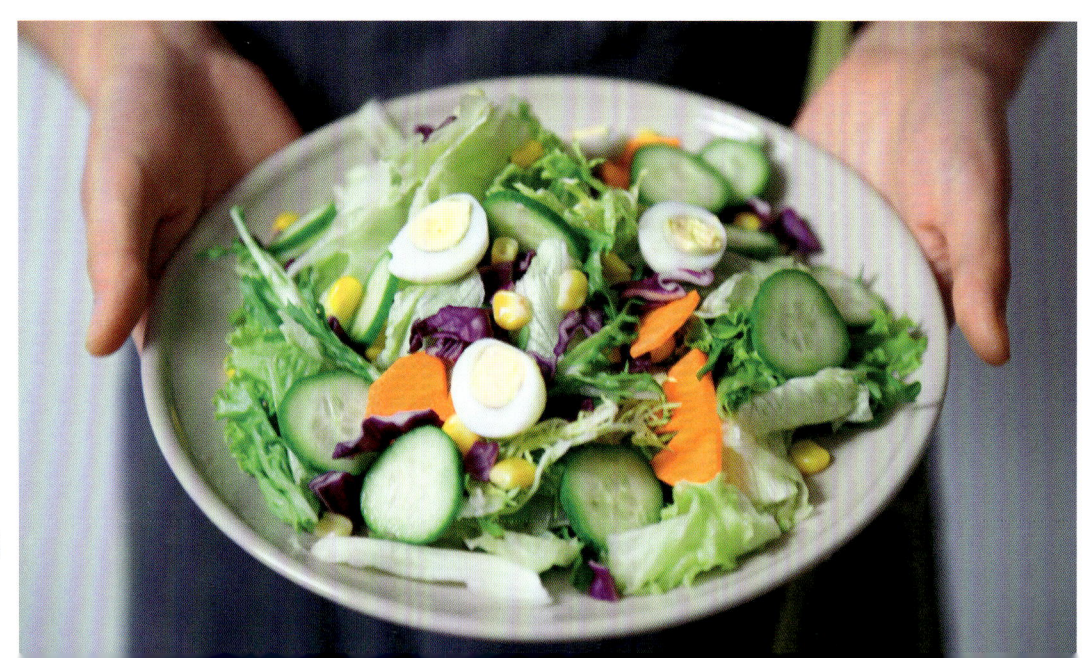

Mid-afternoon snack — if hungry!

Straight after lunch carry on with your Nibbles™. Remember that you have to eat to lose weight, but you are now eating the right type of food to help you shed the unwanted pounds.

Mid-afternoon carry on with your Nibbles™ PLUS a drink and if hungry, eat a small portion of protein such as a tablespoon of cottage cheese or a piece of chicken.

Evening meal and evening snack

Evening meal	- Any protein from the list on page 100 - Grill, barbecue or dry fry foods with fat free spray, NEVER deep fry foods - Choose two vegetables from you list (see page 99) - You could have a thin, unthickened gravy as a sauce - You could use your butter allowance on your vegetables - An organic yoghurt as a 'sweet' and one of your fruits from your daily three fruit 'allowance' - **Start your Nibbles™ again after your meal**
Evening snack	Continue with your Nibbles™. If you're hungry, eat extra protein i.e. cottage cheese, fish, egg, chicken, cooked meats with a small salad.

Continue with your Nibbles™ until bedtime, making sure to have some protein such as a spoonful of cottage cheese, or stock cube size piece of meat or a quarter of a boiled egg, just before bed. This ensures your metabolism will keep working while you are asleep, helping you lose more weight.

Remember your exercises which should be completed morning and evening. They help tone up your body as you lose weight. Remember to prepare your lemon or lime water for the following day.

Tips:
- Avoid cooked root vegetables on the diet
- If hungry, eat a small amount of homemade soup before each meal, then wait wait for ten minutes before eating your meal. This will help you feel full and satisfied sooner

Chapter Nine
Getting active

Gently does it

According to the NHS (**https://www.nhs.uk/Livewell/fitness/Pages/whybeactive.aspx**), people who do regular activity have a lower risk of many chronic diseases, such as heart disease, type 2 diabetes, stroke, and some cancers.

Research shows that physical activity can also boost self-esteem, mood, sleep quality and energy, as well as reducing your risk of stress, depression, dementia and Alzheimer's disease.

'If exercise were a pill, it would be one of the most cost-effective drugs ever invented,' Dr Nick Cavill, a health promotion consultant.

There's no doubt that keeping active has health benefits, but I know from my years of helping PCOS sufferers that physical activity can be a massive challenge for some. If someone is very overweight just moving around the house can be a problem. And if, because of hormonal imbalances associated with PCOS you're suffering with mood swings and/or full-blown depression; then the thought of even going outside can be overwhelming. So, when someone suggests taking up daily exercises or going for walks; it can be really intimidating – something you just don't want to even hear about. That's all perfectly understandable and the reason why this chapter is about encouraging you to try and improve your fitness; slowly, gently and without any pressure.

In this chapter

Start with a good night's sleep

Metabolism boosting exercises

Fat burning exercises for better weight loss

Start with a good night's sleep

Getting a good night's sleep is essential for all of us but if you're battling something as difficult as PCOS, it's even more important.

Simple tips like going to bed earlier, switching off mobile phones and TVs and taking a warm bath can all help towards a good night's sleep. But my favourites are:

- **Get into the habit of going to bed an hour earlier than your usual bedtime**
- **Sprinkle lavender essential oil onto your pillow — it promotes a deeper sleep; you'll be amazed how much better you feel in the morning**
- **Yoga deep breathing or other forms of relaxation exercises also help to relax you and help you sleep**

Gentle exercise

It is important for all PCOS sufferers to participate in some form of gentle exercise. The exercises in this book should be performed in the morning and before bed. These eight special exercises are gentle and non-strenuous and can help you to sleep more soundly. Please note, PCOS sufferers should avoid weights or muscle toning exercise.

Easy Exercise Plan

The exercises on the following pages should be done first thing in the morning, before food and after drinking your lemon/lime water (see page 102).

Please repeat them last thing at night.

The exercises are important because, as you lose weight, they can help to tone up your body.

Always consult your doctor before taking any form of exercise.

Gentle exercise, for example such as walking or swimming, is better than no exercise at all.

Exercise only within your own capabilities. Exercise is more comfortable with knees slightly bent and feet apart.

Before you exercise, gently warm up your body by walking around for three minutes, then you can begin the exercise. If at any time you feel any pain or feel dizzy, you MUST STOP.

Start by breathing in deeply and slowly exhale throughout the movement.

Carefully follow the directions for each movement.

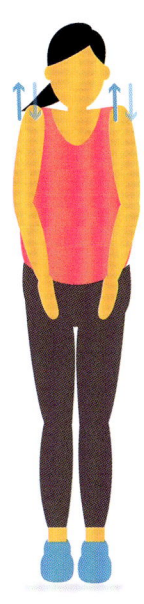
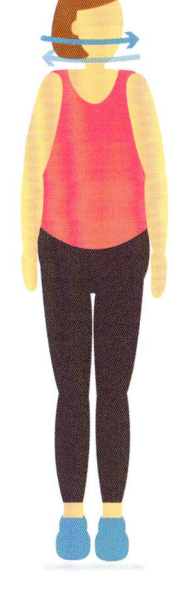

1. Mobilise shoulders
Keeping your back straight and knees bent, gently lift both shoulders and release. Repeat 8 times.

2. Mobilise neck
Keeping your back straight and knees bent, gently turn your head to the right, to the left and take your chin to your chest. Repeat 4 times.

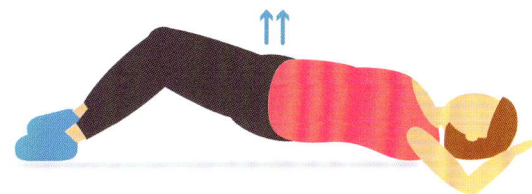
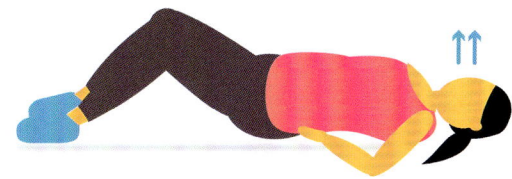

3. Pelvic tilts
Keep your lower back flat to the floor or on a bed. Slowly lift your bottom off the floor, hold for 5 seconds, and release. Try 2 sets of 10 daily.

4. Neck tilts
Keep your lower back flat to the floor or on a bed. Gently lift your head up off the floor, and release. Try to keep your chin off your chest. Try 2 sets of 10 daily.

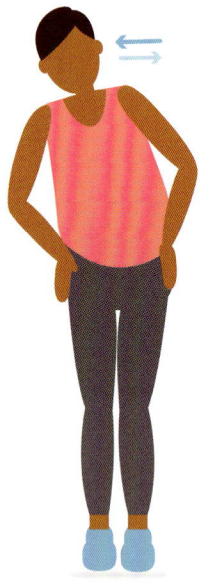

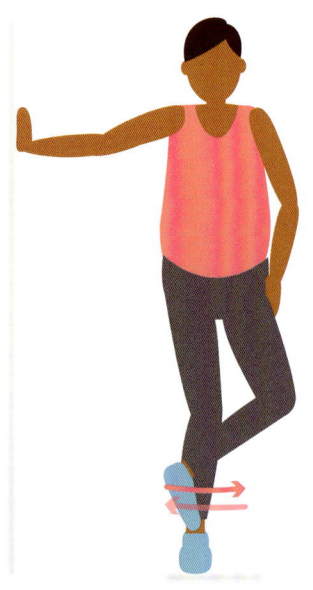

5. Mobilise waist
Keeping your back straight and knees bent, gently lean over to the right, then to the centre, and over to the left. Repeat 10 times daily.

6. Abductors — inner thigh
Push your leg past the centre line of your body whilst keeping your supporting leg slightly bent. Try 2 sets of 10 daily.

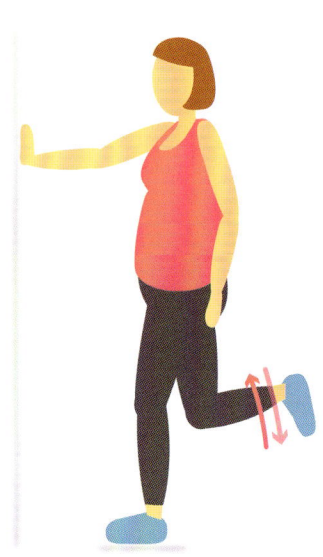

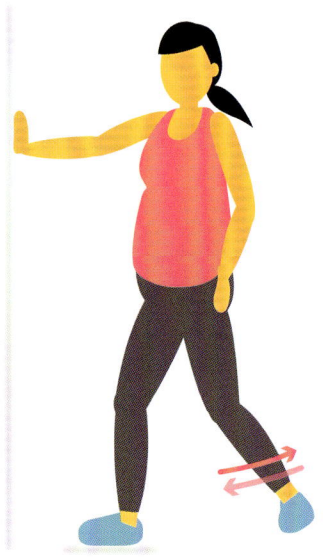

7. Hamstring curl
Working the back of your thigh, lean onto a wall, keeping your supporting leg slightly bent. Do 2 sets of 10 repetitions on each leg daily.

8. Abductors — outer thigh
Gently push your leg out slowly and then down slowly. Try 2 sets of 10 repetitions on each leg daily.

Fat-burning exercises to improve weight loss

If you can manage it, it's important to do some fat-burning exercise, preferably first thing in the morning when your body is in 'fasting-mode' (when your body has not had food for several hours, which is usually first thing in the morning).

Start with five minutes of exercise each day, three times a week, and then gradually build up to twenty minutes a day, every day. For those who find eating a breakfast a problem first thing in the morning, you will be surprised by how easy it is to eat, after a few minutes exercise.

Twenty minutes of brisk walking, jogging (if you are fit enough), cycling, swimming, aerobics, rowing machines, ski-walking and aqua aerobics have all been proven to work well as fat-burning exercises. The reason that these exercises are best performed on an empty stomach is that the low levels of insulin seen first thing in the morning allow your body to access your body fat for energy to be burned by your muscles. After you eat, even a small amount of carbohydrate, your insulin levels will rise. For PCOS sufferers, fat-burning exercises work better on an empty stomach.

If you don't fancy jogging or brisk walking first thing in the morning, you could get on an exercise bike or work through an exercise DVD. It all helps to get you moving. Please remember that if you are not used to exercise, start slowly and work up gradually. You will definitely feel the benefit, very quickly. You could even do your Nibbles™ or Burns™ whilst exercising, and what a difference that will make.

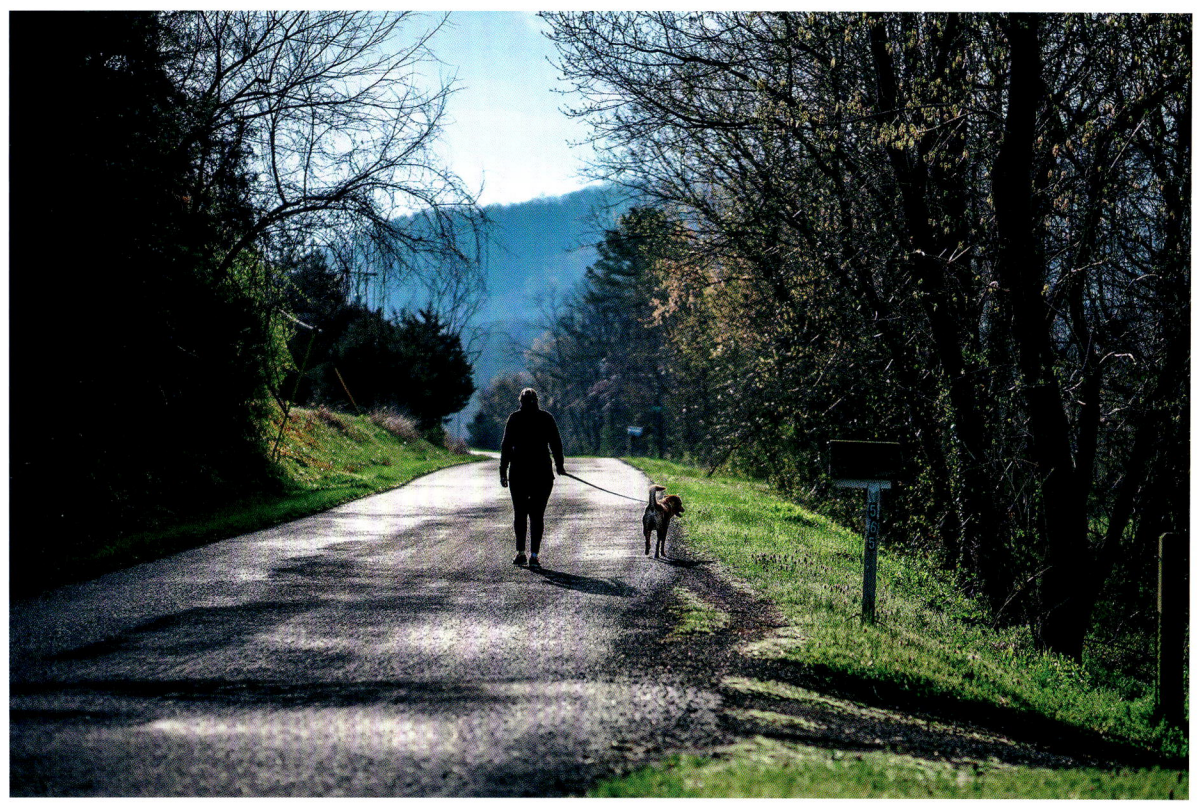

Did you know?

Putting on weight if you have PCOS can increase your chances of developing diabetes. Losing even eight percent of your excess body weight can dramatically reduce PCOS symptoms, as well as helping to safeguard against diabetes and other medical conditions. It is thought that women with PCOS have a different metabolism to other women. It seems PCOS sufferers burn calories at a different rate and store fat cells more efficiently, thus making it harder to lose weight.

The importance of varying your food regularly cannot be stressed enough. Your body gets used to the same food very quickly. Varying your food will 'jolt' your system and help you to continue to lose weight. One of the reasons why eating your Nibbles™ or Burns™ is so effective for weight loss is because it can speed up your sluggish metabolism and help you to lose weight without feeling hungry.

Whether you wish to lose weight to become healthier or to give yourself a better chance of having a baby, my Healthy Eating and Lifestyle Plan for PCOS is tried and tested and has been very successful with thousands of PCOS sufferers.

'In 2015, I was 11 stone 7 lbs and only 5 ft tall. In 2016 I was 8 stone 7 lbs, having reached my ideal weight on the PCOS plan.'

Joanne, Manchester

Chapter Ten
More Life changing success stories

Sharing to help others

On the following pages you can read just a handful of the thousands of success stories where PCOS clients have followed my plan to reduce their symptoms and in some cases, to achieve their dream of motherhood.

Sasha and Andy McDonnell who first led me to find an answer to PCOS, head the line up of generous souls who tell their stories, 'warts and all' so that others, some very isolated and confused by their PCOS condition, can see that they are not alone.

Their hope is that you will be inspired by their success on the plan and never give up hope. They are living proof that there is an answer to PCOS; and one that only requires that you follow the guidance in my Healthy Eating and Lifestyle Plan for PCOS.

> **In this chapter read 'warts and all' stories from:**
>
> **Sasha**
>
> **Andy (Sasha's husband)**
>
> **Cheryl**
>
> **Melissa**
>
> **Emma**
>
> **Jean**
>
> **Sonia**
>
> **Sue**
>
> **Helen**
>
> **Hazel**
>
> **Pat**
>
> **Mary**

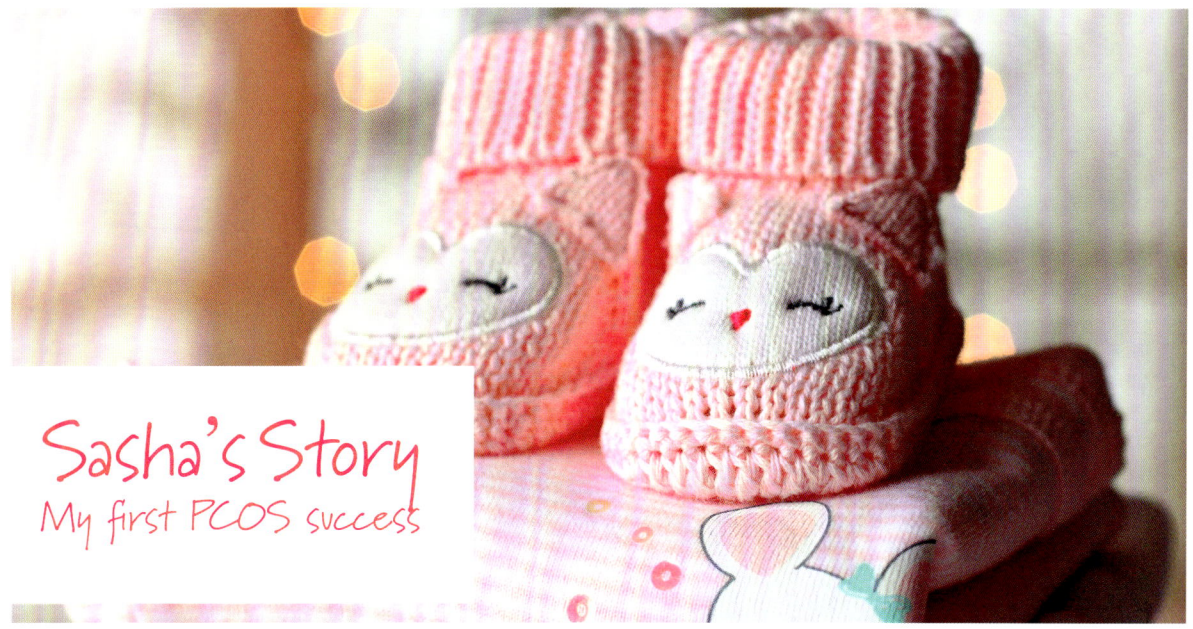

Sasha's Story
My first PCOS success

My name is Sasha, I suffer with PCOS and battled it for thirteen years before I met Norah. I'd tried every diet fad, pills and treatments to reduce my symptoms but nothing worked.

I was infertile, struggled with my weight and suffered depression and the heartache that being childless brought. I was Norah's first PCOS success story.

By the time I was fifteen I had embarrassing facial hair. The kids at school just made fun of me. My periods were every six weeks and the doctor put me on the Pill. Within three years; I was four stone heavier. Hardly going out, I hid myself away.

> 'One day in desperation, I shaved my face. I was so happy — FINALLY!!! the hair was GONE!!!'

One day in desperation, I shaved my face. I was so happy — FINALLY!!! the hair was GONE!!!'

By the next day, my joy had turned to despair – I didn't know it would grow back coarser and darker. Since then, I had a daily ritual of shaving my face. I felt less of a woman and struggled with relationships.

By the time I was twenty-one I weighed 16 stone, suffered extreme mood swings, acne, oily skin, skin tags and aching joints — all the symptoms of PCOS. I was finally diagnosed and referred to a consultant, who was rude and not empathetic in any way. He told me; **'Lose weight, go home and accept you will never be a mother.'**

I was distraught, I rang my mum in tears. It was hard for my family knowing how to support me as I was the only one in the family with PCOS. My own mother had had four children and never experienced any problems.

The heartache years

Eventually, I met and married my husband Andy. We went through the most horrific thirteen years of heartache. We blamed each other, we argued a lot and making love became a chore.

Endless ovulation kits, negative home pregnancy tests, IVF treatments, many scans and ovarian drilling, piled on the pressure. Through it all we were caught up in a continuous cycle of faint hope that always led to devastation.

'Unless you've been through it, no-one really understands the desperation of wanting a child.'

I spent a lot of time crying during those years. I didn't know anyone else with the condition. I felt alone, a freak, and every doctor I'd ever met promised to help, but nothing worked.

It just wasn't fair. Why me? Since I was a little girl, playing with my dolls; I thought I would be a mother one day. Unless you've been through it, no-one really understands the desperation of wanting a child. Andy deserved to be a father, he is an amazing, supportive, loving, husband who adores children and had bonds with family children and friends' children, I so wanted to give this to him.

It doesn't matter who has the problem, it still hurts both of you. Men suffer too but often they have to bury their feelings not wanting to cause further upset or confrontation.

I used to think maybe my husband could be with someone else and achieve the dream of fatherhood.

It was hard watching family and friends having children. Even seeing a stranger's pregnancy bump was upsetting. I couldn't go to birthday parties for my friends' children or christenings either. And, we lost many friends because they felt uncomfortable around us when they became pregnant.

Fate takes a hand

After years of looking to others for answers... I decided to try and find my own answers and started to read loads of PCOS books. In one particular book, a tiny line caught my eye... **'PCOS could affect your metabolic rate'** – this stuck in my mind.

Then one day, fate took a hand. I was talking things through with my sister-in-law who worked in the same building as Norah. She suggested that I give Norah's diet a try because Norah's slimmers used to tell her that it really worked.

Intriguingly, it turned out that Norah's diet was designed to boost metabolism; something I remembered from the PCOS book I'd read.

Shock and disbelief

To be honest, by the time I came across Norah, I'd already become a total non-believer in diets. I was convinced hers would be just like all the rest of them.

Nonetheless, because she focussed on boosting metabolism I decided to try the plan for one month. I also decided that if this one didn't work I'd seek counselling for acceptance and try and focus on the good things I had in my life.

No one was more shocked than me! I lost 7 lbs in the first week of my diet.

By the end of week two another 7 lbs had come off. I was still suspicious…I honestly thought the scales were wrong! But then I noticed my acne had reduced and… I'd not been as tearful or as bloated as normal! And, remarkably, within eight weeks I'd lost an amazing 37 lbs!! My health was starting to improve. I felt so much better and my periods returned.

'No one was more shocked than me! I lost 7 lbs in the first week of my diet'

The pitter patter of tiny little feet

After a few months my periods stopped again. I wasn't worried as I was used to irregular periods. I missed two months which was normal for me. My consultant always advised…'if you don't have a period for two months you need to take some medication to shed the lining of the womb because it can cause problems.'

So, as usual, I had to do a pregnancy test. I duly peed on the stick …and prepared myself for the usual result… in my wildest dreams…I did not expect what happened next….seconds later…to my utter amazement the stick showed positive!!!

The search for answers is over

Through Norah and educating myself I did not realise I was aggravating the PCOS condition by eating certain foods which damaged my health. I'd spent years looking for answers and had never been able to find them. PCOS is not known as the 'nightmare syndrome' for nothing! Before I found Norah that's exactly what it was — A NIGHTMARE!!!

Me and our longed for daughter, 'Libby' born in April 2002

I now know exactly what to eat, but more importantly what NOT to eat to keep me symptom free.

Sasha x

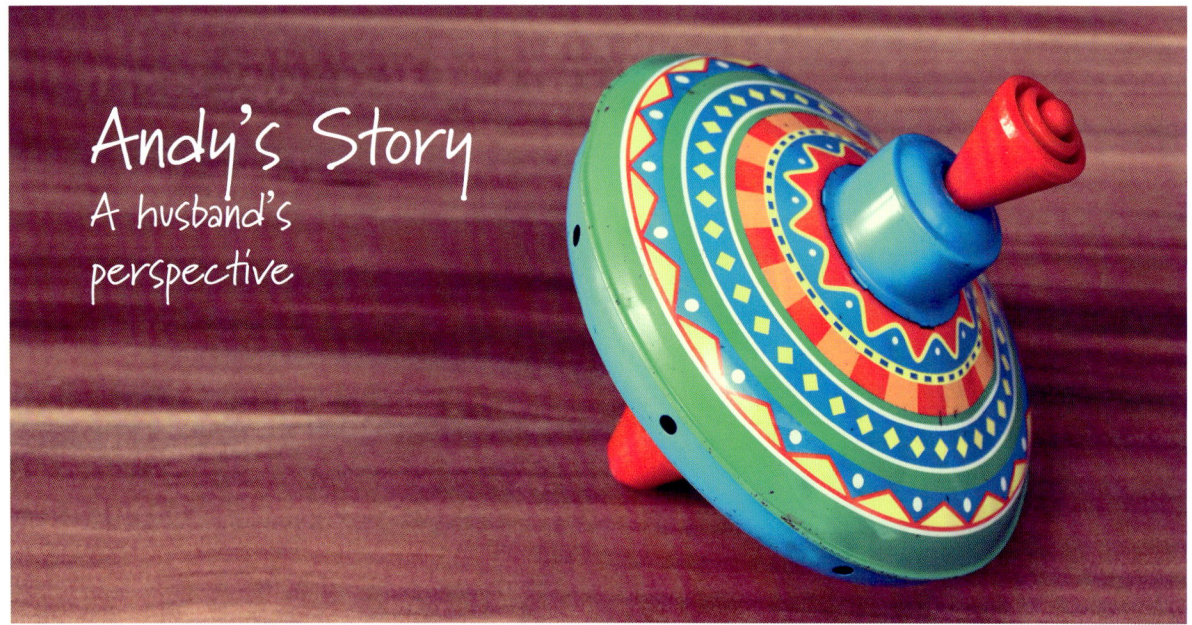

Andy's Story
A husband's perspective

Sasha McDonnell's husband Andy wanted to share his story because, so often, people don't think about what it's like for the husband or partner of a PCOS sufferer. This is Andy's story.

Happy days — but clouds are gathering

Falling in love with my wife was and still is the best thing to ever happen to me. We started courting at seventeen enjoying doing the usual things that couples do. Trips to the cinema, meals out and socialising in the pub.

As our relationship progressed I would buy Sasha takeaway meals and boxes of chocolates which we would both enjoy. It was around this time that she began to put on weight and we put it down to 'being comfortable' in our relationship.

We didn't think at the time; but why didn't my weight increase too?

The first of many crushing disappointments

A few months in to the relationship our love was blossoming and then we were given some fantastic news — Sasha was pregnant! We were both a bit apprehensive but were nonetheless, overjoyed. We became inseparable.

Months passed and our excitement grew. Then one day, I found Sasha in agony with stomach pains. She was rushed to the hospital and later that day we received the devastating news that Sasha had had a miscarriage.

Sasha finally gets a diagnosis

Weeks and months of upset passed and we both carried on as best we could. But couldn't help feeling incomplete.

By this time we'd got engaged and moved into a new home together. Life was getting better. Although, Sasha's mood had altered. She'd become a little more uptight and would get upset at the smallest thing.

She was also still gaining weight. She began to worry too because she'd not had a period for some months. We decided to seek medical advice.

After consultations with numerous doctors Sasha was finally diagnosed with PCOS. We had never heard of it. What was it? Was there a cure for it?

> 'Despite numerous invites to social events we stopped socializing. I found myself making excuses so we didn't have to go.'

We stopped socialising

By this stage, Sasha's mood had dramatically altered. She had put on so much weight that she began to feel uncomfortable with her body and would hide in clothes despite my still telling her how beautiful she was. I meant it but no matter how many times I tried to convince her she seemed to think that I was just saying it to make her feel good.

By now, my wife's depression and ill health had taken a turn for the worst. We'd got married and moved into a new home, but the struggle wasn't over.

Despite numerous invites to social events we stopped socializing. I found myself making excuses so we didn't have to go.

I had to suffer in silence

Watching the one you love having to live with this condition has been so hard. I have had to bury so many of my own feelings. I felt I could never tell her about them because it was difficult enough for her as it was.

I felt like an outsider at times. I could never fully relate to the condition, the symptoms and the many days of depression.

> 'Seeing what PCOS did to her mentally and physically has been emotionally draining at times.'

Deep down I knew she thought she was failing me as a wife. I also knew that she hated not being able to provide me with a child, but I was in love with her and this did not matter to me.

Watching the woman I love suffer was so hard. As long as we had each other, I never contemplated being with anyone else. Why would I? I loved her regardless.

It's been hard watching the woman you love change literally, overnight. The slim woman becoming a curvier one. But it didn't matter, I never found her less attractive. What's inside was more important to me. That's what attracted me to her in the first place.

Seeing what PCOS did to her mentally and physically has been emotionally draining at times. I would try and comfort her, reassure her, but felt I was not being heard. Sasha would shout that I should leave her and find someone else!

It can cause many marriages to fail. There were many trips to the hospital for infertility tests in the hope of becoming parents.

Blaming each other, whoever has a problem, is not great. But I saw it as a shared problem; Sasha did not have to do this alone. I was not going to abandon her.

But trying to convince her was hard, she felt I would be better without her.

The idea of someone else being able to provide me with the child with say a one night stand, was too much for her to bear. She'd often shout at me to leave and find someone else. I would hide my emotions, fears and tears away from her; she was going through enough.

A last gasp attempt at parenthood

Years passed. We were truly in love. We tried to conceive and had our hopes disappointed with further miscarriages.

Finally we decided on a last gasp attempt to become parents by embarking on a course of IVF treatment.

Sasha's weight and health had now started to have a real impact on our lives. She'd developed facial hair, and was mortified, embarrassed. I loved her and accepted the fact she had to shave each day. It was part of the condition she was suffering.

By this time Sasha's weight and devastating PCOS symptoms were affecting her mobility she decided she was leaving me. Doing everyday tasks had become more laboured. I started to feel seriously frustrated and angry. Why had my wife become so ill. Was I doing or helping enough? Our relationship was always strong but I found that Sasha had become distant towards me. Had I done something wrong?

It was then after a heart to heart she informed me that if the IVF did not work; she was leaving me so I could be with someone whom I could father children with.

She called me all the time at work, crying her eyes out. I was devastated. Why was I being pushed away? I totally understood her frustrations, but I knew I only ever wanted to be with her, no matter what.

Despite some false starts, IVF failed. Sasha became even more reclusive and unwell. Things were spiralling out of control and it was now affecting my work.

> 'She informed me that if the IVF did not work then she was leaving me so I could be with someone whom I could father children with.'

Our physical relationship was affected too. It was heartbreaking getting call after call at work from my wife crying telling me she did not want to carry on.

Now it was my turn to cry

I found myself sobbing too. How could things go so wrong all I wanted was to love and care for my wife? We were both so very desperate by now. Not only had Sasha's weight increased to dangerous levels, her symptoms had become more severe she couldn't wash herself, she would stay in bed with pains, her moods became less tolerable what else could we do?

I was beside myself with worry about how ill my wife had become. About how desperate and helpless she had become. Both our families whilst being supportive could not comprehend the full impact PCOS had had on our relationship.

At last a massive stroke of luck

But a chance call was about to change our life forever. A lady called 'Norah' had just set up, offering her diet programme from a room at my sister's beauty salon.

Slimmers were coming and going saying how good the diet was and how they were losing weight. Encouraged by my sister, Sasha decided to try and went along for a consultation.

> 'Living with a woman with PCOS is very hard on the man too. Many years on, I am so grateful to Norah for her dedication and commitment to PCOS women and husbands like myself.'

She was given a diet to boost her metabolism and much to our amazement it started working.

Sasha had begun to lose weight gradually and her health slowly began to improve. Her periods became more frequent until one day a miracle happened.

Our prayers are answered

Thursday had begun like any other we decided to go shopping together, we got the usual two or three pregnancy kits that we would buy — Sasha had missed a couple of periods but that was nothing unusual...it had became a ritual to test just in case.

It was a form of mental torture but we always clung on to hope that one day our dreams and prayers might be answered. We arrived back from shopping and Sasha jokingly waved the tester in her hand 'what if this was positive?'

She then went upstairs as I made us a drink. After a few minutes Sasha returned crying uncontrollably. She could not even speak. She just slid the tester towards me and ran out of the kitchen. To my bewilderment it read positive. I was overcome with all sorts of emotions... was this a mistake?

Glad to say that, after a few nervous, yet joyful months my dreams had come true on 17th April 2002, we were blessed with a daughter, Libby Eva.

Living with a woman with PCOS is very hard on the man too. Many years on, I am so grateful to Norah for her dedication and commitment to PCOS women and husbands like myself.

It is hard to fully appreciate what PCOS can do to a woman. Believe me, sometimes, living with the woman who has the condition can be very trying. I hope my story has helped you see how it does affect both the woman and the man.

As a husband it is hard to stand by and watch PCOS destroy the one you love. I hope you do not let it do that to your wife or loved one. If you are struggling like we were, then you've come to the right place; Norah's diet plan for PCOS is life changing – it has given me and Sasha a family, helped Sasha with her symptoms and **made our once impossible dreams, come true. Thank you Norah!**

Andy x

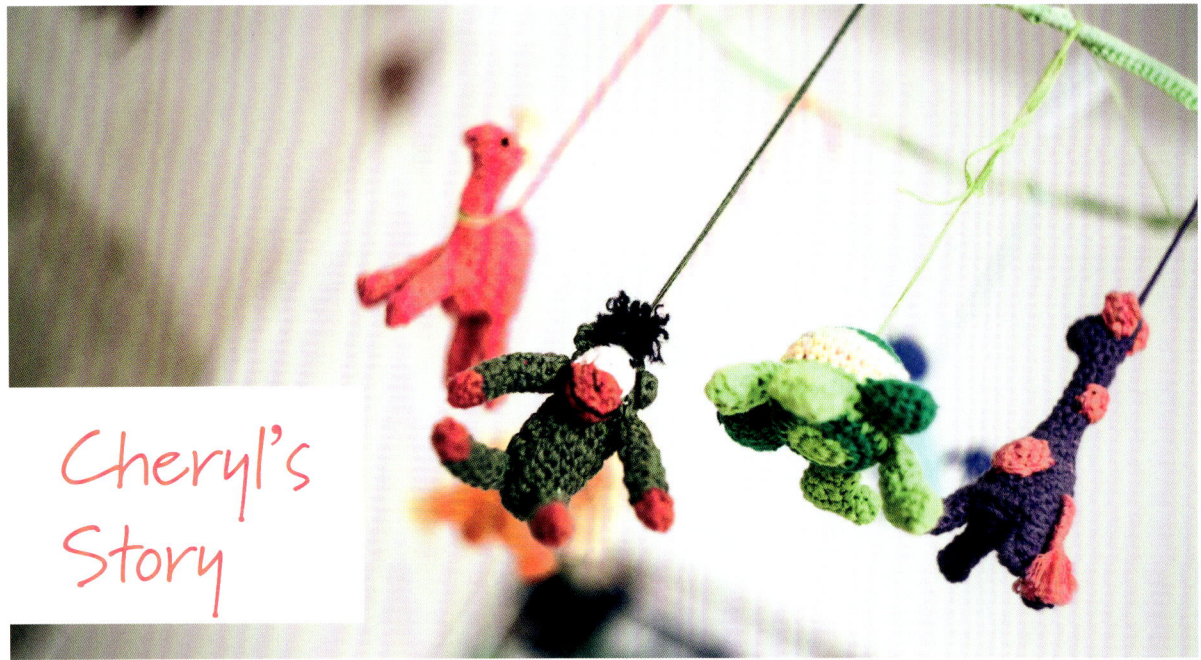

Cheryl's Story

Thinking back on my life and the misery my PCOS caused me made me realise the nightmare started in my early teens. I was thirteen when I started my periods. Not knowing any different, I accepted the dreadful period pains, each month.

After about six or seven painful, heavy periods, they stopped for a few months.

Two years later… my periods were still very painful and irregular. I'd put on a considerable amount of weight and I was suffering with mood swings, excess facial and bodily hair and getting depressed.

The doctor put me on the Pill to regulate my periods and told me to try and lose some weight, suggesting the weight was causing my irregular periods. He didn't want to know when my mother reminded him that when he first saw me at thirteen, I was very slim and yet I still suffered irregular periods. The Pill didn't help – I just gained more weight.

Battling my weight

No matter what diets I tried, I just could not lose the weight. I even starved myself one week, only to find, I'd gained two more pounds.

My mum was always there for me. We tried every single diet on the market. We even tried living on fresh fruit and vegetables. Even though I was only fifteen, I visited all the slimming clubs in the area, but the weight was so stubborn, it just would not come off.

I even tried slimming pills, which I now realise was a silly thing to have done, but I was desperate. I did lots of exercises and I would lose about two pounds, but the following week, the weight was back on again.

My symptoms got worse the more weight I gained. At thirteen I weighed just 8 stone and was 5' 4" tall, which was lovely and slim. By seventeen – I'd soared to 12 stone but I was still only 5' 4" tall.

Needless to say, my confidence had gone and I was even more depressed.

Hiding myself away

I stopped socialising with friends, because I felt everybody was looking at me. I dropped out of college because I just could not cope with the mood swings and increasing amounts of body and facial hair.

By the time I was 18 years old, I was having to shave every day, which was very embarrassing. If I missed shaving, the 'stubble' and re-growth on my face was very unsightly.

There was no constructive support. I was advised to take more exercise. This was ridiculous because I'd been going for long walks every day and went to four exercise classes a week. By the time I was nineteen I'd reached 13 stone.

My depression and symptoms had become so acute, that I just stopped going out altogether. I had no friends, except for the lady next door, (Mrs. Freeman), who was elderly. I used to go in and read to her every day because her eyesight was very poor.

Then...along came Peter!

Peter used to visit Mrs Freeman every week. It turned out, that Mrs Freeman was Peter's grandmother.

He was grateful for the time I spent with his grandmother and used to thank me for taking the trouble to go in and read to her. We started talking and he didn't seem to notice my huge size.

He just told me I was very pretty and we started dating. Or should I say, seeing each other at home, because I would not go out. I was not wallowing in self-pity, I just felt very insecure and knew, in my heart, that something was very wrong with my body.

Peter and I got married when I was twenty-one. We wanted a family immediately, but I knew, at my size, with my non-existent periods and other symptoms, that this could be a real problem.

Discovering I had PCOS

After three years of trying for a family, I went back to the doctor. It was a different doctor who was a lot more understanding.

I explained that Peter and I wanted a family, and told her about all the symptoms I had experienced since the age of thirteen. She thought I could be suffering with PCOS.

This was the very first time that I'd heard of PCOS. I had no idea what it was. My doctor arranged an ultrasound scan. At last something was being done about my health problems. It took two months to get my scan. Yes, I had PCOS. I had a hormone imbalance and this could be the reason for the weight gain and my other symptoms. The scan showed six very large cysts on my ovaries.

The doctor explained that PCOS can, in some cases, cause infertility and in extreme cases, the cysts could become cancerous. There was a strong possibility that I could never have children.

Living with no cure

My doctor said little was known about PCOS, but that I definitely needed to lose weight. She made an appointment for me to see the hospital dietitian. All the dietitian could say was… 'well you seem to be eating healthily, so there is nothing more I can suggest'.

> 'All the dietitian could say was "well you seem to be eating healthily, so there is nothing more I can suggest…".'

At the age of twenty-five I had just been told I had PCOS, I could never have children; and that I had to cope with my symptoms as best I could. I was devastated. I had suffered with health problems since I was thirteen years old and had experienced twelve years of misery. I can remember coming out of the surgery, after this consultation, and breaking my heart crying, in the car. Tears were rolling down my cheeks — I felt that my life was over.

As you can imagine, this made me even more depressed and my relationship with Peter started to become very strained. I did not feel like a 'real' women. I never wanted the physical side of the marriage, because I felt fat and ugly. And my skin problems and acne were much worse by this time.

The nightmare continues….

Peter was so understanding, but this did not seem to help. I went into a real depression. All we both desperately wanted was to have a child of our own, but there seemed to be no help available.

I scoured the Internet, looking up every piece of advice on PCOS. I joined support groups on the Internet because I would not go out. All the information seemed very conflicting and very complicated. Even the support groups could not give me any diet advice. All that was available was support from other sufferers, swapping different ideas, most of which I had already tried.

Another visit to my doctor resulted in her putting me on metformin. Unfortunately, it caused me to have really bad side effects; I was constantly feeling sick and had very bad headaches. My PCOS symptoms did not improve, nor did the frequency of my periods.

Longing for a child

I was taken off metformin and after a while was put on clomid but it made me dizzy and light-headed. I was 27 years old when my doctor suggested IVF treatment, but insisted that I lose weight before she would start any treatment.

By starving myself and exercising in my bedroom, virtually round the clock, I did manage to lose 14 lbs in three months. I started IVF treatment, which worked, but, unfortunately, I had a miscarriage at six weeks.

As you can imagine, this was a real blow and my depression came back.

By the time I was 29, Peter and I were drifting apart and I decided I needed to talk to my doctor again. My doctor suggested counselling for my marriage problems and perhaps consider adoption. Peter and I decided it was an excellent idea.

We had all the visits from the adoption agency, went through all the paperwork and did all we could to proceed.

Too fat to adopt!

All Peter and I really wanted was a baby, of our own, to love and cherish, forever. Unfortunately, yet again, this ended in failure. We were informed by the Adoption Society, that, because of my obesity, I was a health risk. They knew about the PCOS, but the decision had been made and I was rejected. Yet again, another bitter disappointment.

> 'We then thought about fostering a child, but were given the same advice. "You are obese, and we feel it inappropriate to place a child in your care".'

We then thought about fostering a child, but were given the same advice. 'You are obese, and we feel it inappropriate to place a child in your care.' One agency actually said, 'If you were looking after a child and had a heart-attack because of your weight, what do you think would happen to the child?' I was devastated again, yet another blow.

Bingeing to console myself

Because of all these upsets, I just could not stop eating. My weight was increasing week by week. I had now given up all hope of ever losing weight and becoming a mum. I was on antidepressant medication from my doctor and, by this time, Peter and I were hardly speaking.

It was not Peter's fault. I had gone into a shell because I knew it was my fault that we could not have a child. After all, I was the one with the PCOS.

In December 2002, I was watching a programme on the television about childless couples and I turned to Peter, after the programme had ended, and said 'I think we should get divorced, I cannot give you children and you are still young enough to find a partner who can'.

Peter was so upset, he came over, put his arms round me and said 'I love you Cheryl, it doesn't matter about having a family. All I want is you'. I thought this was a wonderful thing to say, but I really did not believe that he meant it.

The TV show that changed my life

Then it happened. And everything started to change for the better. We had Christmas and New Year holidays and I made a New Year's resolution to try, once again, to lose weight. I thought to myself... 'I did get pregnant once, even though it was with IVF, and I can do it again. I will just have to keep trying with my diet'.

It was fate that took a hand. On January 13, 2003, Peter had come home early from work for his evening meal and was sat in the living room with the television on, at 6 pm, watching the news. I was in the kitchen when I heard this terrific scream from Peter: 'Cheryl come in here quickly, hurry, hurry, hurry'.

He was watching the BBC News and there was a lady called Sasha, who had suffered with PCOS for more than 15 years. She had lost weight on a special healthy eating and lifestyle plan. Sasha had lost weight quickly, but the best news was that she had conceived, naturally, and had given birth to a baby girl, called Libby, the previous April.

Sasha explained…'after years of trying I'm finally losing weight, and my symptoms are reducing! I was able to understand, for the very first time, what I was doing wrong and what I should be eating'.

After getting all the details from the TV company I started on Norah's plan that Sasha had followed and lost 5 stone in six months. My weight had gone up to nearly 18 stone and now I was down to 13 stone.

Everything begins to improve

For me, more important than the actual weight loss, was that my PCOS symptoms were reducing. My facial hair was getting finer and my curly hair, which had been falling out because of the PCOS, started to become much thicker again. My mood swings too became much less frequent. After I lost 4 stone, I had a period for the first time in years.

The best news ever happened when I went back to my doctors for the result of another ultrasound scan. She was delighted with my weight loss, but then told me that the ultrasound scan had shown that my cysts had dramatically reduced.

> 'Several PCOS support groups advise their members to take a look at this diet and I do know that three of my friends with PCOS also lost weight on it and felt great.
>
> 'Only other PCOS sufferers, like those who read this book, could possibly understand how I now feel.'

I'd had six large cysts at the beginning, but there were only two showing on the scan and those were shrinking. My doctor advised me to keep doing what I had been doing and was delighted with my progress. My confidence started to come back and I found I had a renewed, positive outlook on my life.

My doctor advised her other PCOS patients about my diet and the success I was having.

Several PCOS support groups advise their members to take a look at this diet and I do know that three of my friends, with PCOS also lost weight on it and felt great. Only other PCOS sufferers, like those who read this book, could possibly understand how I now feel.

Cheryl x

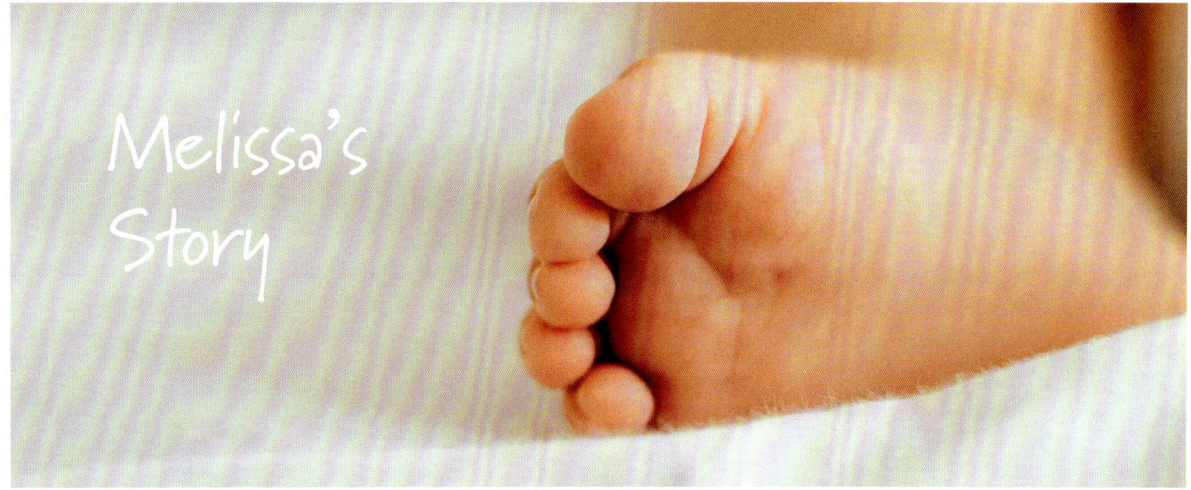

Melissa's Story

'Melissa Atherden (age 31) had severe PCOS and desperately wanted to have a family. Following my Healthy Eating and Lifestyle Plan for PCOS helped her to achieve her dream.

'When Melissa looked in the mirror all she could see was a depressed, obese woman covered in dark, thick, coarse facial and bodily hair. Every day, she had to shave, like a man.

'She also had 'cyst-like' spots covering her entire face and neck. These spots required antibiotics to help to clear them. Her skin was very oily. She suffered severe mood swings, dizziness and painful, flooding periods. She'd endured all these physical problems for years and they'd taken their toll on her. To put it mildly, she was fed up with life and did not know which way to turn for help.

'Melissa had had seventeen years of hell and there was nobody there to help her. The final straw came when her consultant told her that she could never have a baby. She was so shocked, she cried for days.'

Norah xx

Melissa – my story

I have suffered with symptoms since I started my periods at eleven years of age. I visited doctors many times over the years but had to wait until I was 28 before I was diagnosed with PCOS.

For years I was left to suffer with horrendous, heavy periods and stomach cramps. I sometimes fainted with the pain. I suffered with sickness, and, at a very young age, I had to regularly take strong painkillers, to ease my symptoms. I would curl up in bed with two hot water bottles – one on my stomach and the other on my back. I had to sit in a very hot bath to numb the pain. I regularly had time off school because of severe symptoms. Sometimes my periods were so heavy I could not leave the house.

At fourteen, after suffering for three years, my doctor prescribed the Pill, which didn't help.

My mother asked for specialist help but was refused. When I was twenty-eight I literally begged the doctor again for help. That was when I was sent for an ultrasound scan and PCOS was diagnosed. I was told one in six women suffered with this condition and that I was one of those with severe symptoms.

It was explained that it can result in infertility and in some rare cases could be cancerous. One consultant told me; 'It is very unlikely you will ever conceive'. I was devastated.

> 'When I was 28, I literally begged the doctor again for help. That was when I was sent for an ultrasound scan and PCOS was diagnosed.'

Typical student meals

One of my many symptoms was severe weight gain. From age 18, when I was at university, I started to gain a terrific amount of weight. I missed a lot of lectures because of being so ill. I was eating pasta and the usual student foods without realising that these were the foods to be avoided, especially when you suffer with PCOS. Because nobody would diagnose what was wrong with me, I had no idea what to do or what to eat.

At one stage I stopped eating, thinking that this would help me lose weight, but it didn't; I just became very tired and depressed.

My facial and bodily hair was very dark and coarse. It was costing me a fortune to regularly remove the hair...in the end I had to resort to shaving. It was a total embarrassment because the more I shaved the thicker the hair became. When I was out, people used to comment on my appearance and stare at me so I stopped going out.

My weight soared to over 16 stone. I tried every diet I could think of Weight Watchers, Slimming World, Slimfast, Zone diets, Heart Foundation diets. I would lose 4 lbs and then put it all on again, plus a few pounds more. Nobody believed me when I said I was sticking to the diets, but I really was. It seemed the less I ate the more weight I gained. When a size 20 outfit became too tight, I just refused to buy 22s. I felt so ugly and unfeminine.

As you can imagine, by now depression had started to set in. I felt so different to other people. I was overweight, infertile and suffering with facial and bodily hair. I realised there was something very seriously wrong with me when my periods finally stopped altogether. I couldn't understand why, even though the periods stopped, the pain and all the other symptoms were still there. I visited my doctor for help, but again I was ignored.

> 'It was costing me a fortune to regularly remove the hair...in the end I had to resort to shaving.'

Meeting Ed

A few years later I met and married Ed, a computer engineer. We desperately wanted a family. After trying, without success for some considerable time, my doctor finally agreed to refer me to another specialist, who confirmed that severe PCOS was the problem.

I was told that the chances of my having a baby were very slim. At best, the specialist said I had a six percent chance of conception. The medical profession was very vague about what else I could do to help myself, just kept telling me to lose weight.

I had been trying to lose weight for years, even starving myself and all the specialist said was; 'when you suffer with PCOS, your metabolism is different and it is very difficult to lose weight'. Coming out of the surgery, I broke my heart crying. I was told to come back in six months and they could discuss various fertility treatments or other options.

I was offered fat loss drugs, but when the severe side effects were explained, it was not an option that I wanted to try. What could I do now? I felt that life was too much to take. Even walking down the street people would stare, point fingers and comment on my appearance. 'I'm sure that they think I just sit at home and binge all day, but I don't. It's so unfair'; I would say to my husband.

Ed knew how hard I tried; we ate the same food. I had much smaller portions than he did, but still gained more and more weight.

Finding Norah...my star was rising

By now I was desperate, and at my wits end. I decided to take matters into my own hands. Whilst I was waiting for my appointment at the hospital, I searched the internet to find out about PCOS.

I found Norah's website for PCOS weight loss. In which in those days was under the name of 'Vitaline'. For the first time I could understand what PCOS was and how it could be treated with a healthy diet and lifestyle changes. So far all the doctors had failed me and Vitaline had been established for over 30 years, so I enrolled.

At last – light at the end of the tunnel

In my first week I lost 7 lbs, eating real food and no gimmicks. I learnt that Norah had spent years working with PCOS support groups, hospital consultants and PCOS volunteers, all in an effort to try and design the very best diet and lifestyle plan to help PCOS sufferers.

My healthy eating plan was so easy and for the first time in my life, I felt I was getting some proper help. It inspired me when I read that Vitaline, Norah's company had helped women to conceive. There were testimonials online to read too and I was encouraged to contact these women and ask them about their personal experiences of using the plan.

I felt wonderful. After three weeks on the plan, I noticed that my PCOS symptoms had started to reduce slightly. I was less moody, my skin was a little clearer, I had more energy, I was not craving food and I felt much healthier.

It was explained to me that when you suffer with PCOS, there are certain foods that your body cannot tolerate and once these foods are omitted and replaced with other healthier options, the weight can start to come off.

Then a miracle happened....

By the time I found Norah I had not had a period for over a year, which was really worrying. Two months after starting the plan my periods returned and they were not as painful. I couldn't believe it. At first I thought it was just a lucky chance...but then I had another period the following month. Now I knew this diet was the one for me. I went to see my consultant and he was impressed by the way I looked and said it was all down to my new diet.

A few months later, I got a big shock. I missed my period and at first I was so depressed because I thought things were going wrong again...but...I felt so well. I took a pregnancy test and discovered that I WAS PREGNANT!

> 'My consultant was convinced it was the diet which helped me lose a considerable amount of weight and that that led to my becoming pregnant.
>
> 'I now know what to eat and more importantly what not to eat. My consultant recommended Norah's diet to all his PCOS sufferers and not just the ones that want to get pregnant.'

I carried on with my healthy eating plan throughout my pregnancy and gave birth to my beautiful baby daughter Mia. My consultant was convinced it was the diet which helped me lose a considerable amount of weight and that that led to my becoming pregnant.

I now know what to eat and more importantly what not to eat. My consultant recommended Norah's diet to all his PCOS sufferers and not just the ones that want to get pregnant.

Sharing to inspire

This plan is definitely the best one for me because after Mia was born, I was so busy, that I went off the plan for a few weeks.

My skin problems, food cravings and tiredness came back very quickly. As soon as I went back on the plan, the problems disappeared again.

I do hope my story will inspire other young women to demand help earlier, because PCOS is a devastating condition and nearly destroyed my life.

I am delighted to write my story for Norah's book because I really do believe that without the help of this plan, I could never have succeeded in losing weight, which reduced my symptoms and helped me become pregnant and give birth to Mia, my beautiful baby daughter.

Melissa x

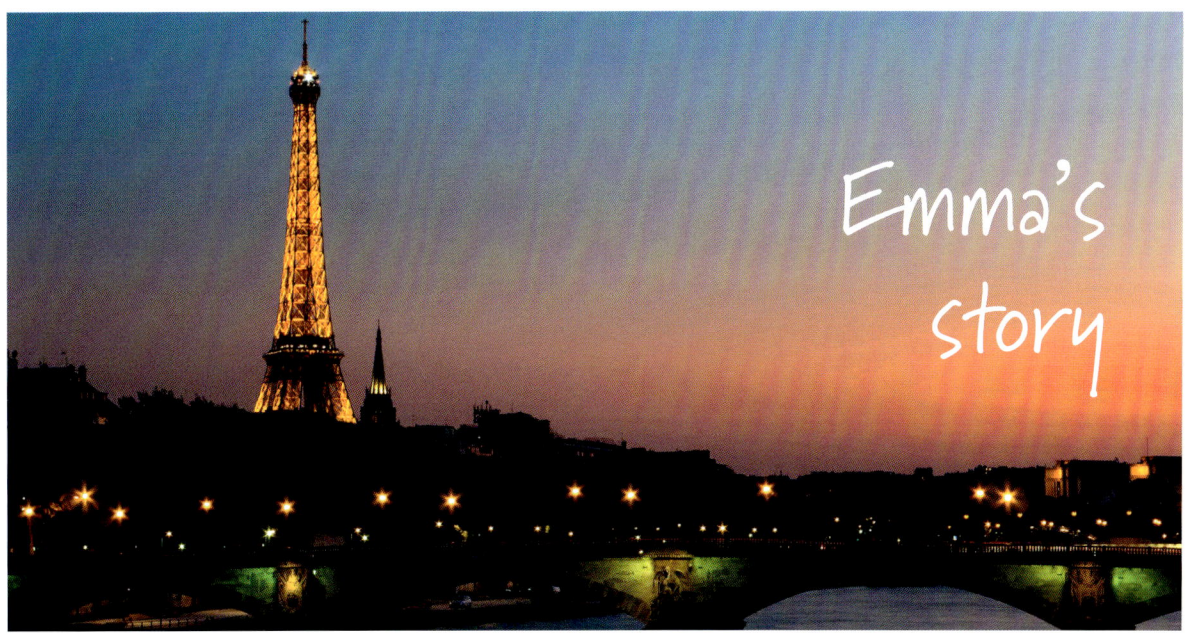

Emma's story

When I first came to Norah's clinic in Manchester, I was 17 years old. My mum, Marjorie was really worried about the amount of weight I'd put on — I was nearly 21 stone!

I am normally a very 'bubbly' person but being so overweight was depressing me. And it got worse. I started to grow facial hair — a complete nightmare.

My mum had tried me on many diets and even cut down my food to very small portions but nothing was working. In fact, I was gaining more and more weight, every week. The good thing was my mum had been one of Norah's slimmers herself and decided that we should try her plan as it had worked for her.

By the time I got to Norah my weight was a major problem. I'd started gaining weight when my periods started. But these were very irregular. Sometimes I'd have a period each month, but then, for no apparent reason, they would disappear for months...but I still got period pains.

My mood was all over the place — it was so upsetting. My mum had taken me to the doctor but all he said was that I should lose weight.

As soon as Norah saw me she said she thought I was suffering from PCOS. Neither me or my mum had heard of it. It was such a relief to think that there was something 'wrong' with me; because at least I could point to something and say that's the reason I cannot lose weight.

Norah suggested we go back to the doctor and explain my symptoms in great detail and ask for a blood test or an ultrasound scan. In the meantime, Norah got me on the PCOS plan. She didn't want to waste any more time and I was happy to get started. Maybe I would be able to go out with my friends again soon!

On the plan I was eating healthy, organic food and learning good eating habits that would help me for the rest of my life. In the first week I lost 8 lbs — I couldn't believe it!

After the first month I noticed my skin was a lot better. All my spots had gone and my acne was really, actually, starting to clear.

Within two months I'd lost 20 lbs and my facial hair was much finer. My energy levels were up and I felt more confident and more able to cope with the condition. After six months I'd lost three stone and my periods came back.

> 'In the first week I lost 8 lbs — I couldn't believe it!'

It was quite a shock. I wasn't expecting a period because I hadn't had one for over a year...and this time...there was no pain. I was so happy. I've had regular periods ever since and all my symptoms are less.

To top it all, I was able to go on holiday to Paris with my friends – something I would never have done before.

For the first time I felt normal. I bought clothes that were on trend and was able to enjoy life like every other young person.

Emma x

> 'As soon as Norah saw me she said she thought I was suffering from PCOS. Neither me or my mum had heard of it. It was such a relief to find out that there was something 'wrong' with me; because at least I could point to something and say that's the reason I cannot lose weight.'

Note: It is essential that PCOS is diagnosed as early as possible. If Marjorie had not brought Emma to me, it could have been many more years of suffering and misery before she would have been diagnosed with PCOS. (Norah)

More success stories

Jean, California, USA

I was desperate for a baby. Three unsuccessful attempts at IVF, severe obesity, mood swings, and tiredness, was causing me to get very depressed. I did not have body or facial hair, but I was irritable, and my husband and I were ready for splitting up.

PCOS and the symptoms it brings, can put a terrific strain on a relationship. I heard about Norah's healthy eating plan and decided to give it a try. The diet is great. I have a good appetite and am never hungry. In fact, the secret of me losing weight and becoming healthy, is to eat small and often. It is an easy to follow plan. I lost 24 lbs in six weeks. Amazing.

Sonia, Wales

I was diagnosed with PCOS when I was 23. I have suffered for two years, getting little or no support from the various professionals. I attended PCOS support groups and was told about Norah Cozens and decided to do the plan.

I wasn't trying for a baby yet, but I did want to get healthy and give myself the best possible chance of pregnancy, for the time when I may decide to have a family.

After three months on the plan, my sugar levels were improving, my excess body hair was going, and my consultant was delighted with my progress.

The diet is low fat, low sugar, low carbohydrate, but high protein. The most important thing I have learned about PCOS, is what I must eat to help improve my health.

I also learned how to take each day at a time, follow my plan, eat all the correct food, particularly the fruits, have the Nibbles™ every 15 minutes and then I just watched the weight go.

I lost 28 lbs on the plan. I was very pleased to feel fitter. I now go out more with my partner, as I feel more self confident.

Sue, England

I conceived naturally and had my first born, a boy in 1992. I went on to have another relationship and married Andrew in 1997. We wanted a child together and a sibling for my son from my previous relationship. We had been trying for five years. I thought the problem must have been with Andy as I had already had a baby.

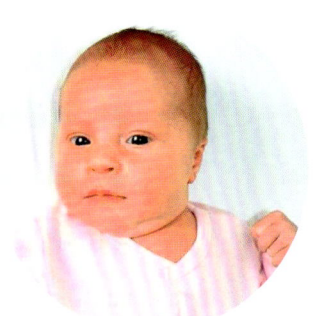

In 2000 I found out I had PCOS. So we had fertility treatment. The first attempt failed but with the second the procedure worked and I was fortunate enough to get pregnant with twin girls, Rebecca and Charlotte. I was so ill from start to end. I was 37 when I had the twins. Our family was complete… or so we thought.

We moved to Dubai for five years. We had no intention of having any more babies. I hadn't used contraception for ten years — there was no need.

I read about Norah's diet and thought wow, I will try this. This was so I could lose weight and feel healthier — **not to get pregnant**! Obviously, I was sceptical but… wow …I started it and did it religiously. I felt so healthy and started having periods but still thought nothing about getting pregnant.

By October I had lost over three stone in four months. I felt amazing. At the end of October I missed a period — bear in mind I was 40 years old. I felt sick in the morning and thought no, I can't be…I am too old. But I did a test and ohhhh my…I was pregnant!

I was shocked and scared. I was 40, oh my God no way! Norah's diet had made me healthy. I also started ovulating again. I felt amazing throughout the pregnancy and gave birth to another miracle baby. Emily was born in July 2006.

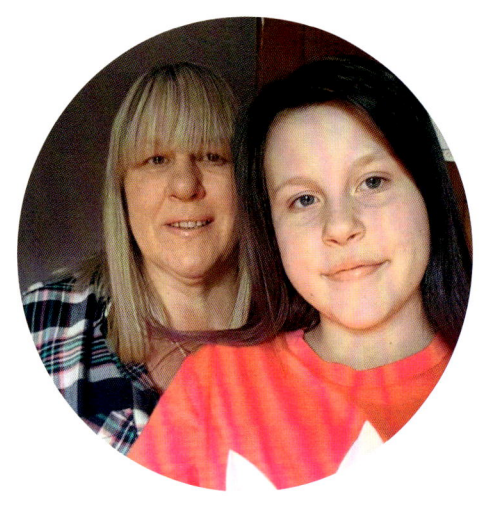

With Norah's diet and the amazing encouragement from the Vitaline team I didn't just feel better because I lost weight (four stone in total), I also had a miracle baby.

'Thank you' Norah for your amazing diet and Sasha for being there for hundreds of people. Please if you have PCOS, try this healthy eating plan — it's amazing and never give up on your dream — never say never.

Helen, Manchester

PCOS can be so physically and mentally draining and the impact on my life was so far reaching and much more so than I actually realized at the time.

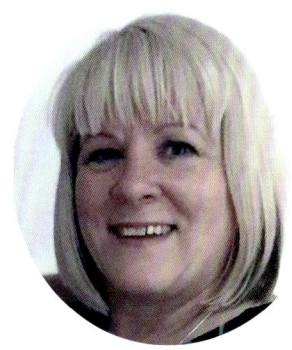

I was diagnosed with PCOS two years after my second child was born, twenty-four years ago. Fortunately, getting pregnant hadn't been an issue for me but the horrific symptoms associated with PCOS commenced with avengence, virtually as soon as my second child was born. Despite following my GP's advice to follow a low GI diet, I was still consistently gaining weight every week.

I was referred to the endocrinology department at my local hospital as I was still gaining an average of 2 lbs per week, had male pattern hair growth (which I hadn't had previously) and my periods had all but stopped but when they did happen, I flooded!

At the hospital I was prescribed the mini Pill (for my periods) and tried metformin (for weight control) for 12 months but neither resolved any of the symptoms and in fact made me feel a lot worse so I gave up taking them.

I met Norah back in 2007 when I had just come out of hospital after having investigations for endometrial carcinoma (PCOS meant I was at higher risk) and my mum read an article about Norah's clinic in Denton and how successful people had been in losing weight.

I weighed in at 15 stone despite eating practically nothing and frantically exercising five times a week in my local swimming pool. I just wanted to feel better, to eat more healthily and have more energy especially as I was working full time in a very demanding job with two young children.

Previous to seeing Norah, it became apparent, that I wasn't eating anything like enough food to sustain my mental and physical health as I had usually eaten all the same sorts of foods and too many carbs!!

On Norah's diet I lost 5 stone and 2 lbs but most importantly have kept the weight off for the past five years. It is still quite incredible to believe that given the amount of food I eat I can still lose weight. Mentally and physically I feel and look like a different person and have so much more energy and zest for life!

I can't promise you it's easy but if your head is in the right 'space' and you are prepared to be well organised and willing to plan ahead you will be successful.

Hazel, Manchester

I regard Norah as a good and true friend. Norah first helped me to lose weight in 1996 and maintain my target weight for a long period of time. At the end of 2004, I was diagnosed with PCOS, and through a carefully controlled diet, planned by Norah, I later conceived naturally and combined with excellent hospital antenatal care, gave birth to my daughter Eleanor in summer 2006. Eleanor was the 110th baby born with Norah's help. This I feel is the greatest gift anyone can give!

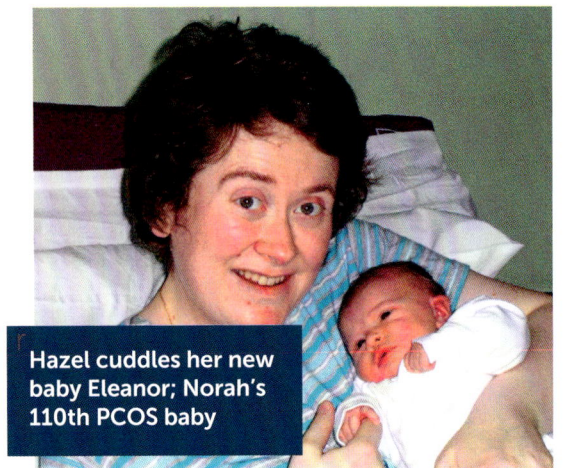

Hazel cuddles her new baby Eleanor; Norah's 110th PCOS baby

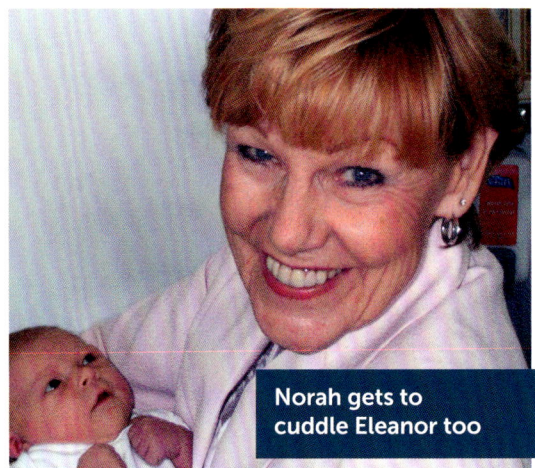

Norah gets to cuddle Eleanor too

Pat, Swinton, Greater Manchester

Being desperate for a baby and having suffered three unsuccessful IVF procedures, I thought my dream of becoming a mum had gone. PCOS ruined my life. I saw Norah on a TV programme, decided it was worth another try.

Within twelve months of starting the healthy eating plan, normal periods returned, I lost weight and became pregnant.

Mary, South London

I have suffered with PCOS for years. I was not overweight, but I was tired, lethargic, suffered with mood swings and could not conceive. I had not had a regular period for four years. I have been on metformin and clomid, for a considerable time, without improvement. My last hope was Norah's diet. It had worked for my friend. After being on the healthy eating plan for just three months, I had my first proper period. I was delighted. I feel healthier and my energy levels are improving.

Chapter Eleven
The Maintenance Diet

Congratulations!

You've succeeded in losing all your excess weight! You've probably climbed a mountain of control and commitment to get here...so it's time to award yourself some gold stars!

Chances are you'll have had mostly good days... but inevitably some bad ones too. That's because it's never easy for PCOS sufferers to lose weight. But you've battled through and won the day — you should be so proud of yourself.

By losing weight you will have increased your general health and very importantly for PCOS sufferers, helped to improve your metabolism.

So now you've made all that effort to achieve your ideal weight, you need to do everything you can to keep it off! And that's not as difficult as you think. All you have to do is follow my Maintenance Diet for PCOS on the following pages.

If you stick to my guidance you will be able to keep your metabolism working well. This is the key to keeping the weight off. No more *yo-yo dieting!*

In this chapter

How to maintain your weight

General hints and tips to keep your weight stable

Your daily allowances

Breakfast options

Snacks and lunch options

Evening meal and evening snack

How to maintain your weight

Things you should do:

- Weigh yourself once a week only

- At the beginning allow yourself ONE luxury a week (maybe a nice, healthy meal out?)

- Try and get a hobby that involves some form of exercise. Now you are slim you may have the confidence to go swimming or join Zumba classes. Walking is good too and burns lots of calories

- If you feel you have cheated a little more than you should have, go back to the original plan for a day or two; doing as many Nibbles™ as you can. Once the unwanted weight has disappeared go back on this Maintenance Diet

- Keep a regular check on what you are eating — it will help to stabilise your weight

- Don't forget — if needed you have my Binge Recovery Guide too!

> If you want to stay slim, healthy and symptom free, then good eating habits are essential and need to be maintained **for life!** An occasional slip will not be a problem but only if it is **occasional.**
>
> Read the Maintenance Diet very carefully and let's face it, when you can have a few cheats every day and still stay slim, you won't want to go on a binge. You'll have the best of both worlds – a slim, trim healthy you, plus a few 'cheats' along the way.

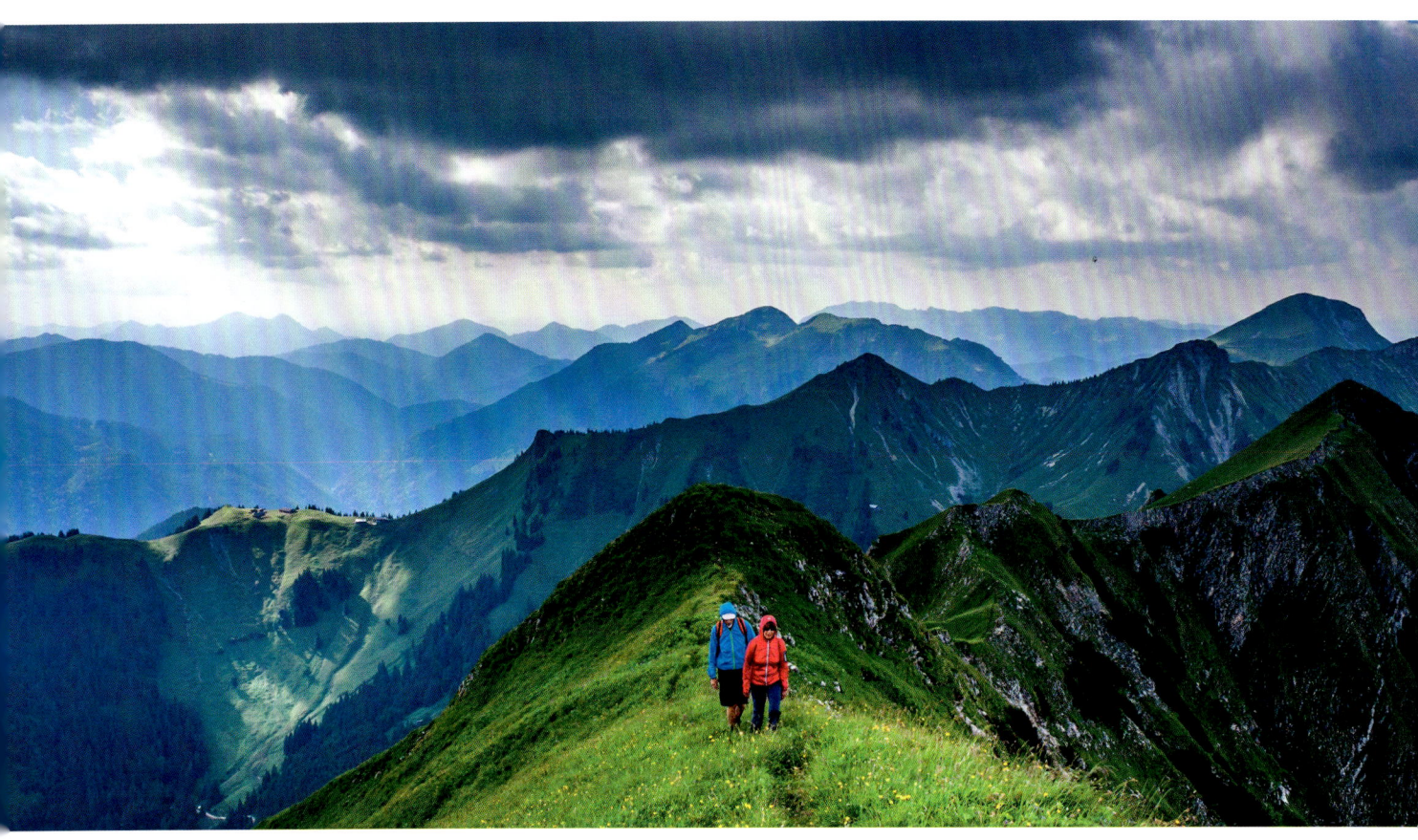

Once you have reached your desired weight, the Maintenance Diet can help you stay slim and boost your fitness levels. As your fitness level improves, you will be able to do more. This might seem a bit ambitious now… but in time you will feel that anything is possible — the sky's the limit!

General hints and tips to keep your weight stable

- Be careful not to miss any meals, eat regularly
- Be sure to have protein with every meal
- Start each day with a cup of cooled, boiled water containing a **paper thin** slice of lemon or lime (before breakfast!)
- Vary your meals as much as possible – choose a different breakfast, lunch and dinner every day
- Drink plenty of fresh water
- Always eat yeast free varieties of bread, or crispbreads – you could be carbohydrate sensitive
- Eat organic where possible
- Avoid additives and processed foods
- Remove excess fat from foods and skin from chicken and fish
- If you feel hungry and are tempted to cheat, have some soup or eat some protein. This could be a dessert spoon of cottage cheese
- Casserole, steam, grill or dry fry your food – never deep fry
- If going out for a meal make sure you use the Guide to Eating Out on page 155
- Avoid microwaving in plastic containers – use glass instead
- Avoid drinking from cans or plastic bottles

Your daily allowances

- 284 ml/½ a pint of full fat milk (not skimmed or semi skimmed)
- 3 pieces of fruit (preferably pears or kiwi)
- 14 g/½ oz of butter OR full fat mayonnaise OR a tablespoon of oil
- 2-3 portions of vegetables
- Plenty of fresh water

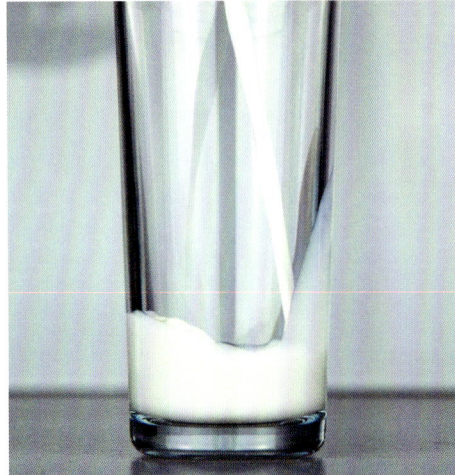
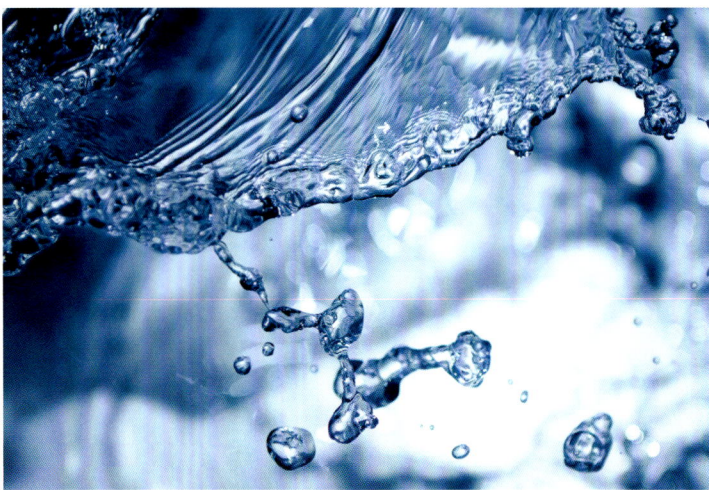
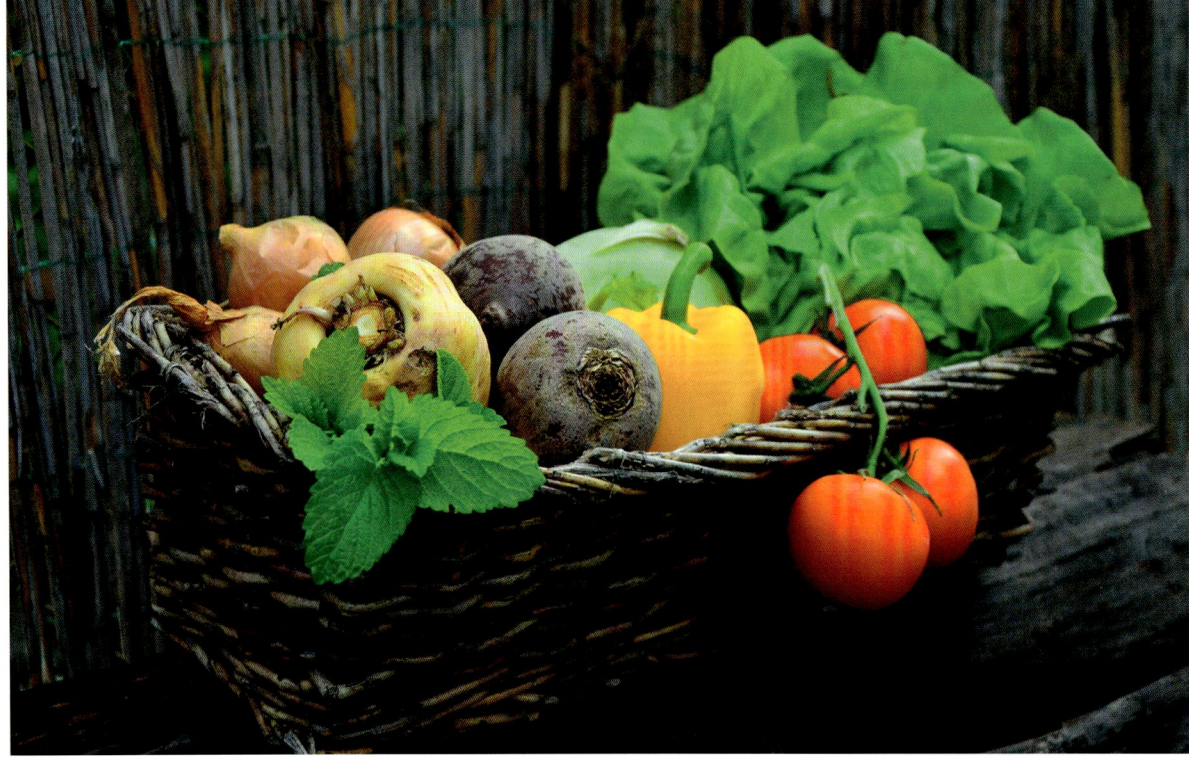

Breakfast options

114 mls/4 fl oz unsweetened fruit juice (not from concentrate)
OR half a small grapefruit or orange

PLUS a choice of ONE of the following:
A small bowl of cereal with a little milk plus 10 berries and ¼ teaspoon of seeds
OR an egg (may be poached, baked, boiled or scrambled)
OR 2 slices of grilled bacon plus 2 tomatoes
OR 1 piece of fish (steamed, baked or grilled – NOT fried)
OR 2 grilled high meat content sausages with tomato and mushrooms
OR 2 pieces of fresh fruit with a tablespoon of natural yoghurt
A crispbread OR a small piece of yeast free bread is permitted with breakfast

Snacks and lunch options

Mid-morning

1 cup of tea or coffee with milk from your daily allowance – NO sugar
PLUS an apple
OR a small plain biscuit
OR a small piece of plain cake

Lunch options (salad can be added to any of these options)

284 ml/½ pint of homemade soup
OR unsweetened fruit juice
PLUS 2 slices of yeast free bread, pitta bread OR rye bread, filled with any meat, poultry, fish or egg
OR a salad with any meat, poultry, fish or egg – 1 small potato can be added
OR a portion of protein with vegetables chosen from the list on page 99
OR 3 crispbreads or rice cakes topped with protein
OR 1 jacket potato plus a filling

After lunch

1 piece of fresh fruit or organic natural yoghurt
PLUS 1 cup of tea or coffee with milk from your daily allowance

Mid-afternoon snack

1 drink PLUS a portion of cottage cheese (any variety) on a crispbread, if hungry

Evening meal and snack

Evening meals

Choose from lunch menu but avoid repeating the same meals

Evening snack (if hungry, but no later than 9.30pm)

A drink of your choice with any ONE of the following:
A small piece of low fat cheese on a crispbread
OR an organic yoghurt
OR a small plain biscuit
OR two crispbreads with a small amount of protein

The above is your guide to your healthy eating 'future'.

Feel free to experiment with foods you like but bear in mind how hard it has been to lose weight. Be careful not to overdo things... otherwise you will find yourself back at square one. Keep up the good work and happy eating!

Chapter Twelve
Easy soups & sweets

Some favourite recipes

Over the years my slimmers have shared some of their favourite soups and sweets recipes.

The soups are a great way to satisfy hunger — eating soup before a meal will make you feel fuller sooner. And, the sweets will satisfy your 'sweet' tooth without sending you off the rails.

The recipes use everyday ingredients that you will be able to find in local stores and supermarkets. I hope you enjoy them as much as we have.

Recipes to enjoy on this diet

Chicken and onion soup

Curry soup

Caulicream soup

Beansprout soup

Asparagus soup

Mixed vegetable soup

Fruit crumble

Four fruit whizz

Apple meringue

ALLERGY DISCLAIMER

Anyone with known or unknown food intolerances or food allergies must take personal responsibility for food choices associated with these recipes.

I will not assume any liability for adverse reactions from any of the ingredients listed in these recipes or any liability for any injuries sustained in the preparation of these recipes.

Soup Recipes

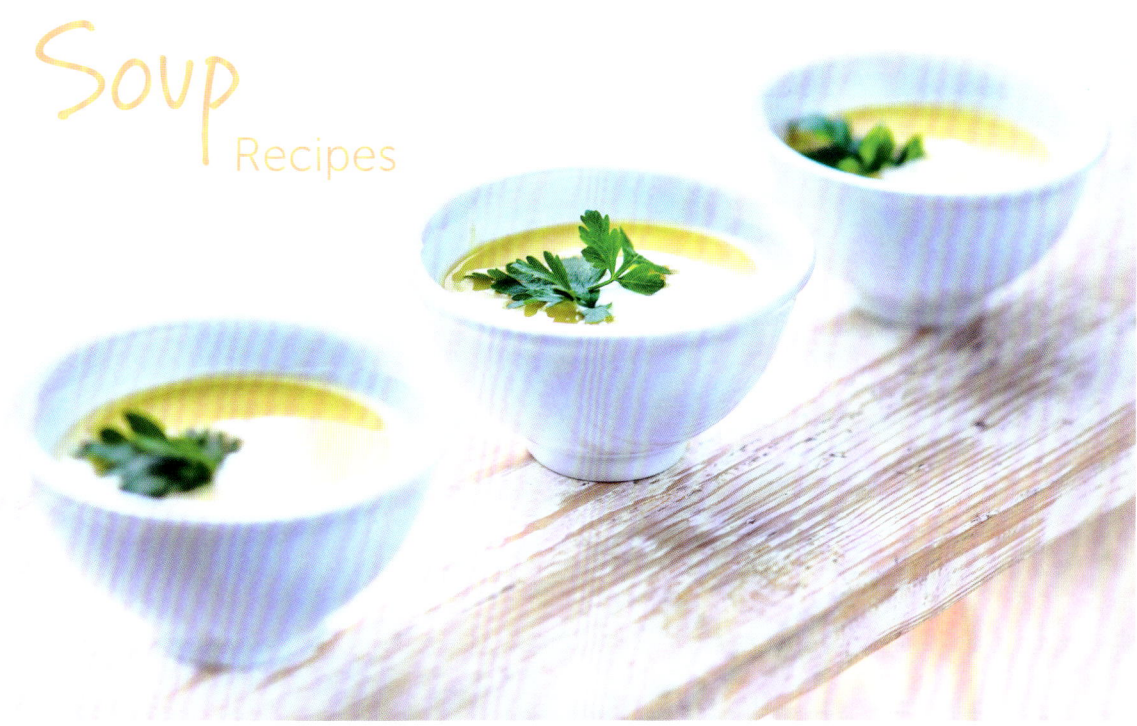

Chicken and onion soup

Ingredients

142 ml/¼ pint of organic milk, 113 g/4 oz chopped onion, 142 ml/¼ pint chicken stock

Method

Simmer for ten minutes. Liquidise or sieve and simmer for a further five minutes. Please add chopped chicken if you want chicken pieces in your soup.

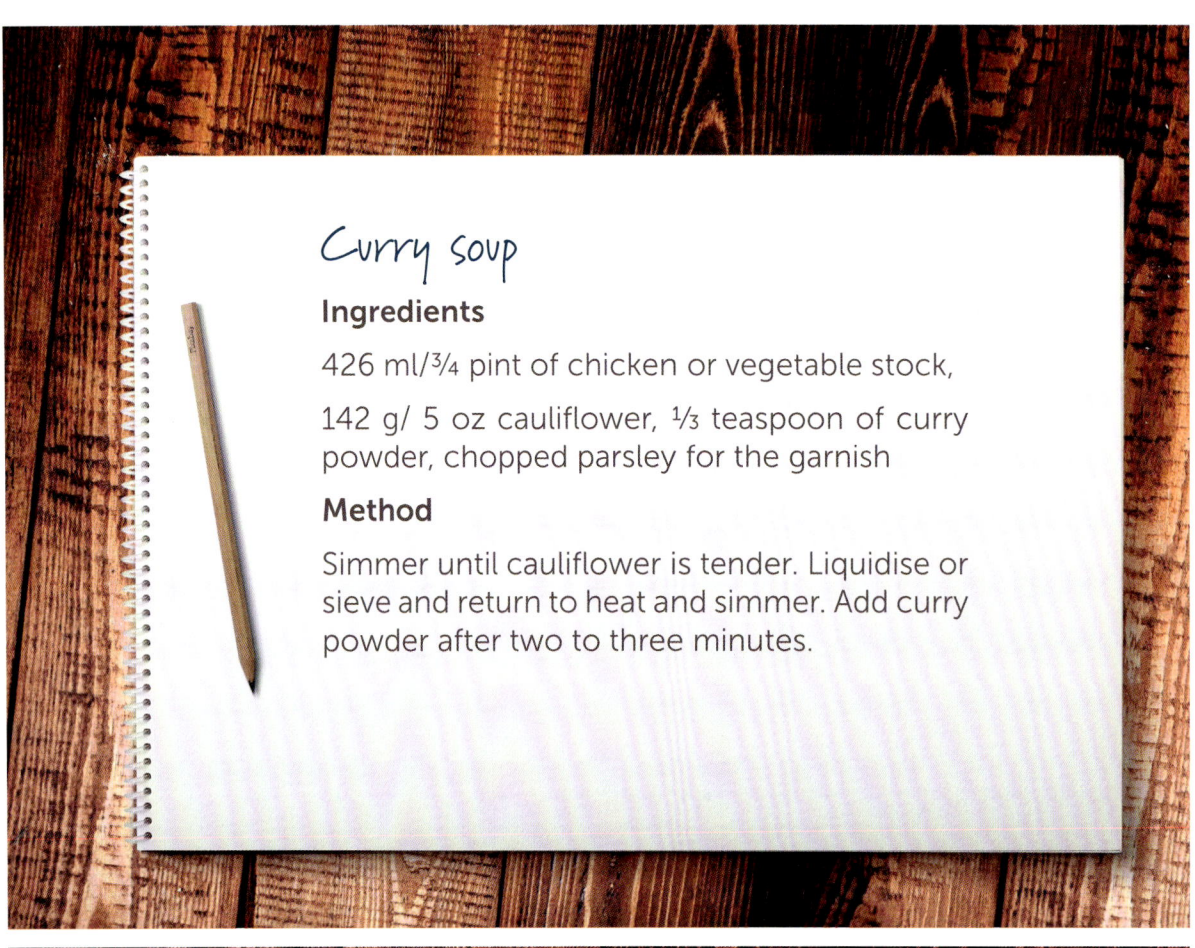

Curry soup

Ingredients

426 ml/¾ pint of chicken or vegetable stock,

142 g/ 5 oz cauliflower, ⅓ teaspoon of curry powder, chopped parsley for the garnish

Method

Simmer until cauliflower is tender. Liquidise or sieve and return to heat and simmer. Add curry powder after two to three minutes.

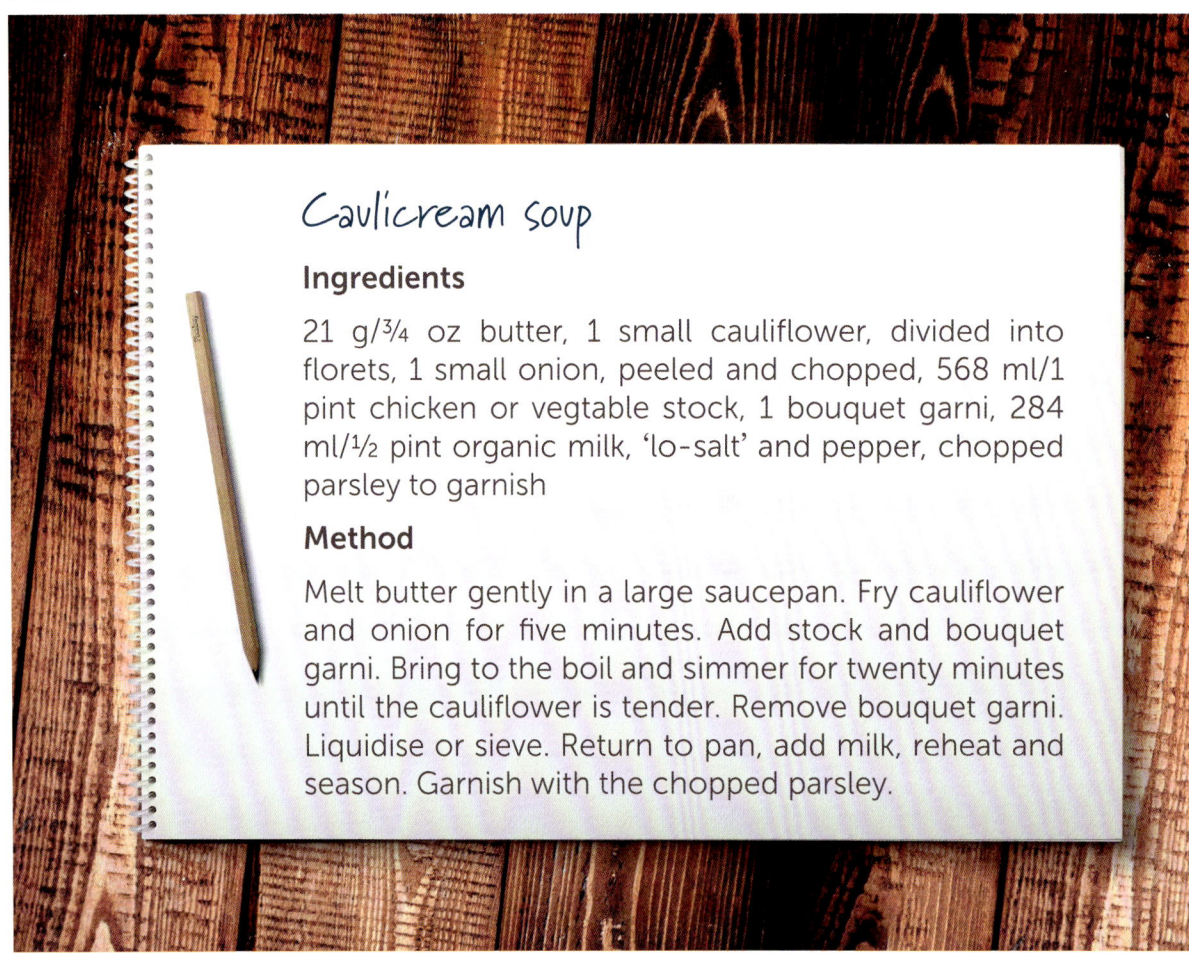

Caulicream soup

Ingredients

21 g/¾ oz butter, 1 small cauliflower, divided into florets, 1 small onion, peeled and chopped, 568 ml/1 pint chicken or vegtable stock, 1 bouquet garni, 284 ml/½ pint organic milk, 'lo-salt' and pepper, chopped parsley to garnish

Method

Melt butter gently in a large saucepan. Fry cauliflower and onion for five minutes. Add stock and bouquet garni. Bring to the boil and simmer for twenty minutes until the cauliflower is tender. Remove bouquet garni. Liquidise or sieve. Return to pan, add milk, reheat and season. Garnish with the chopped parsley.

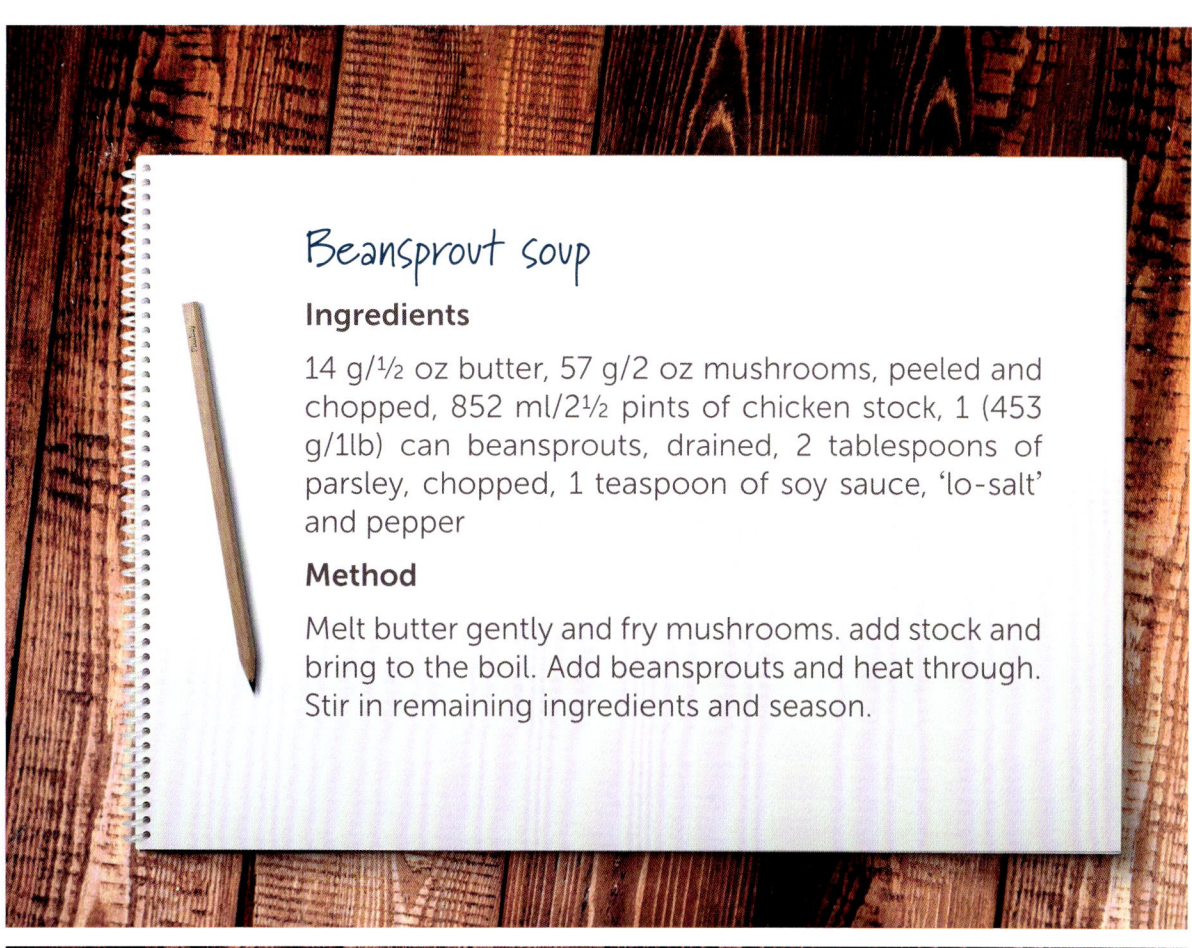

Beansprout soup

Ingredients

14 g/½ oz butter, 57 g/2 oz mushrooms, peeled and chopped, 852 ml/2½ pints of chicken stock, 1 (453 g/1lb) can beansprouts, drained, 2 tablespoons of parsley, chopped, 1 teaspoon of soy sauce, 'lo-salt' and pepper

Method

Melt butter gently and fry mushrooms. add stock and bring to the boil. Add beansprouts and heat through. Stir in remaining ingredients and season.

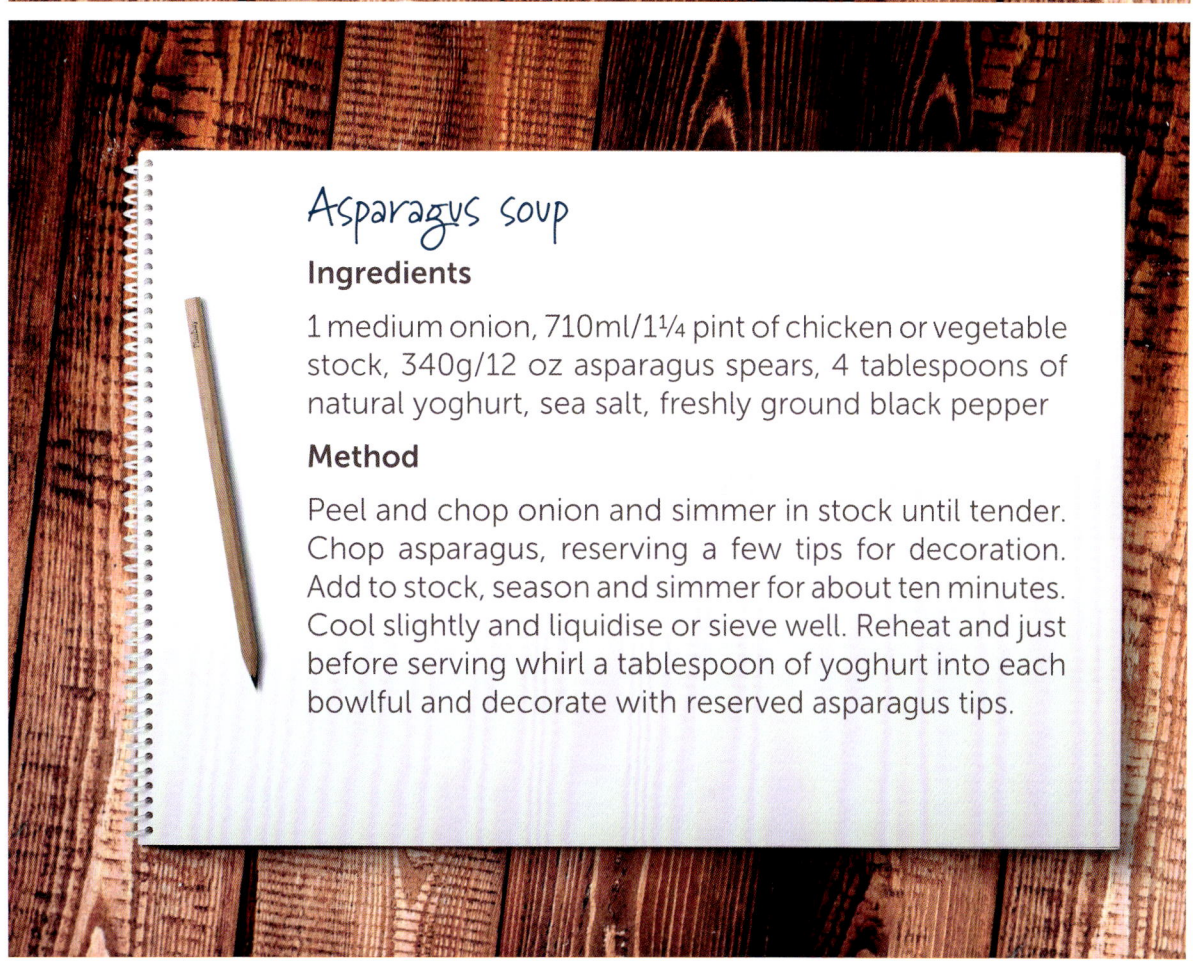

Asparagus soup

Ingredients

1 medium onion, 710ml/1¼ pint of chicken or vegetable stock, 340g/12 oz asparagus spears, 4 tablespoons of natural yoghurt, sea salt, freshly ground black pepper

Method

Peel and chop onion and simmer in stock until tender. Chop asparagus, reserving a few tips for decoration. Add to stock, season and simmer for about ten minutes. Cool slightly and liquidise or sieve well. Reheat and just before serving whirl a tablespoon of yoghurt into each bowlful and decorate with reserved asparagus tips.

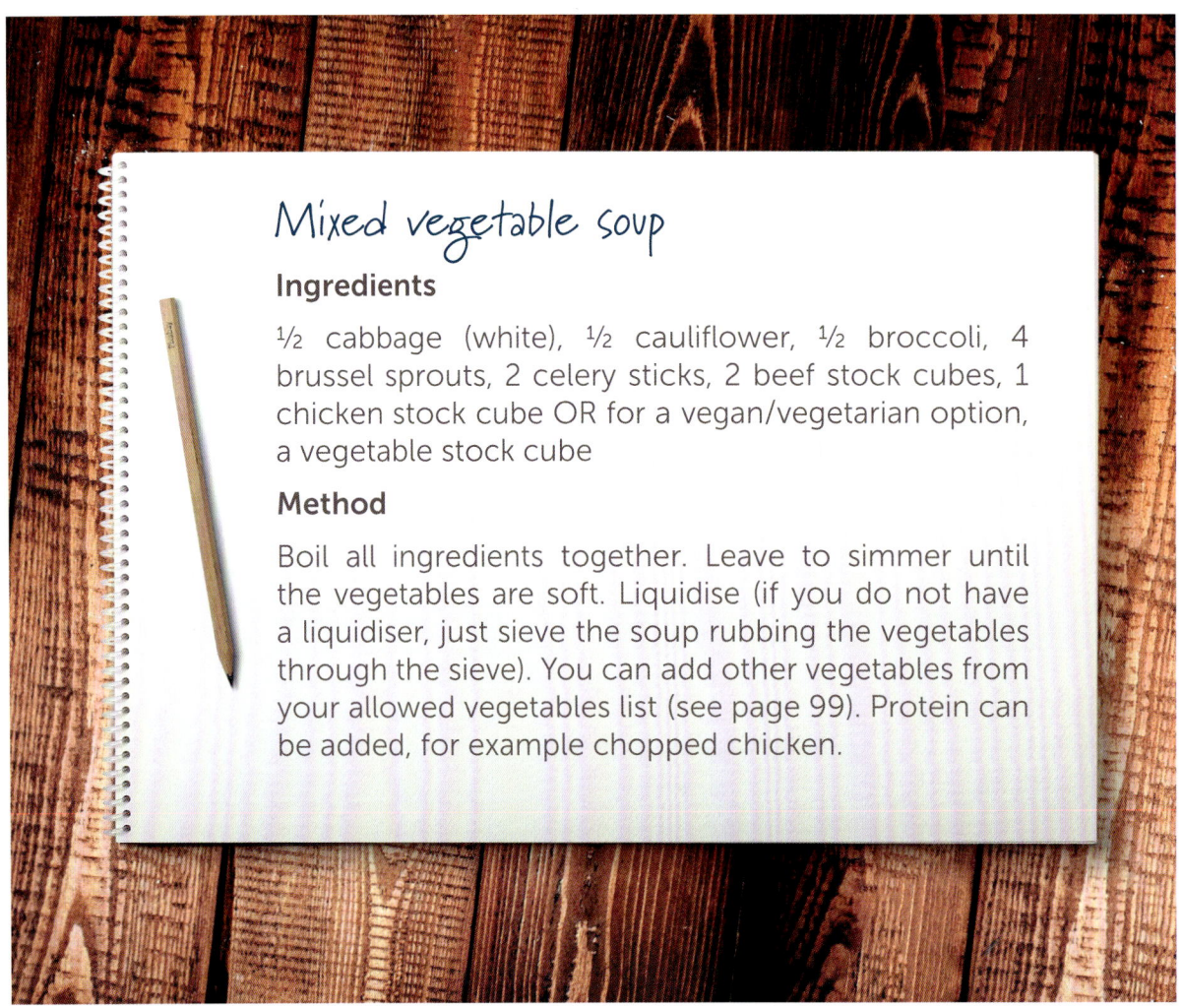

Mixed vegetable soup

Ingredients

½ cabbage (white), ½ cauliflower, ½ broccoli, 4 brussel sprouts, 2 celery sticks, 2 beef stock cubes, 1 chicken stock cube OR for a vegan/vegetarian option, a vegetable stock cube

Method

Boil all ingredients together. Leave to simmer until the vegetables are soft. Liquidise (if you do not have a liquidiser, just sieve the soup rubbing the vegetables through the sieve). You can add other vegetables from your allowed vegetables list (see page 99). Protein can be added, for example chopped chicken.

Remember: Soups are a great start to your meal. If you wait ten minutes after eating your soup and before starting your meal, you will already feel quite full. This will also help to stop you being tempted to eat more or have a fattening dessert.

Sweets
Recipes

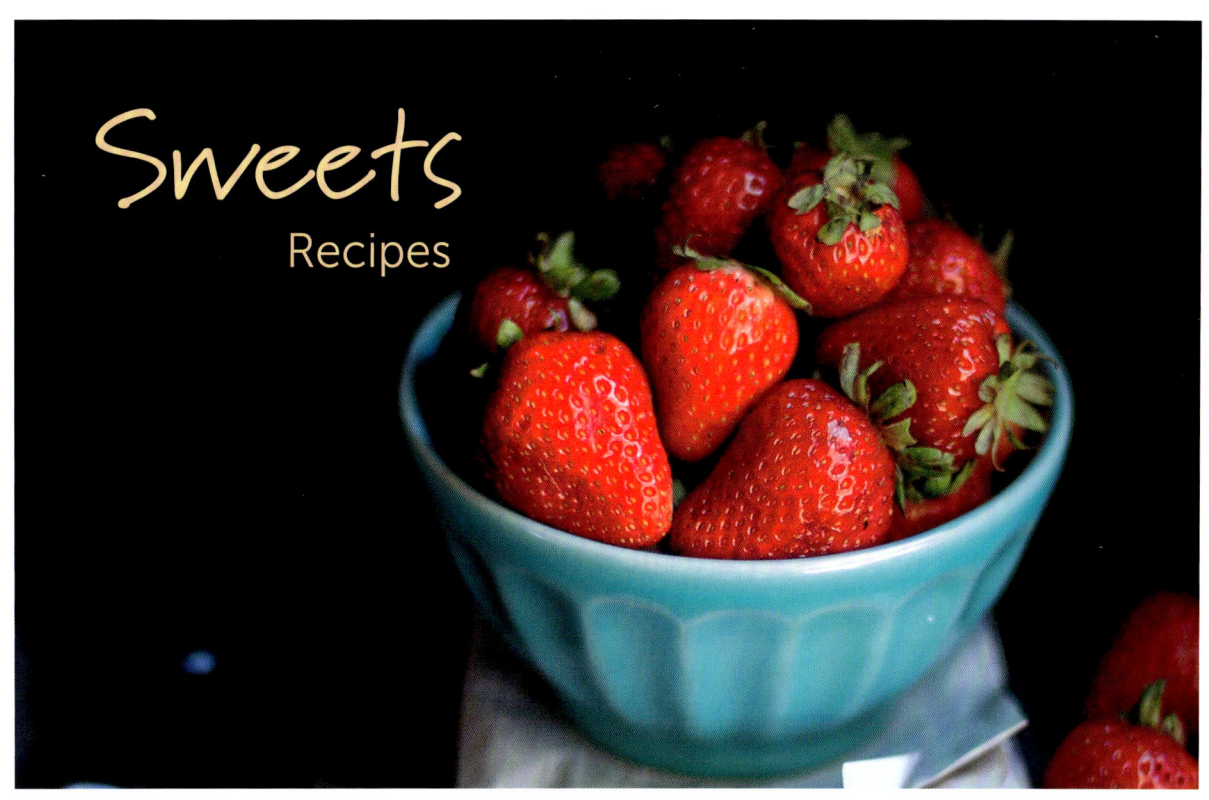

Fruit Crumble

Ingredients

2 apples (rhubarb or pear if you prefer)
Natural bran
3 knobs of butter
Nutmeg

Method

Simmer the fruit in a small amount of water until tender. When cool, add sweetener, if necessary. Place the fruit in an ovenproof dish and sprinkle with 2 tablespoons of natural bran. Add 2 or 3 knobs of butter, a tiny amount of nutmeg if liked, and place in the oven for ten minutes. Cook until crispy and brown on the top.

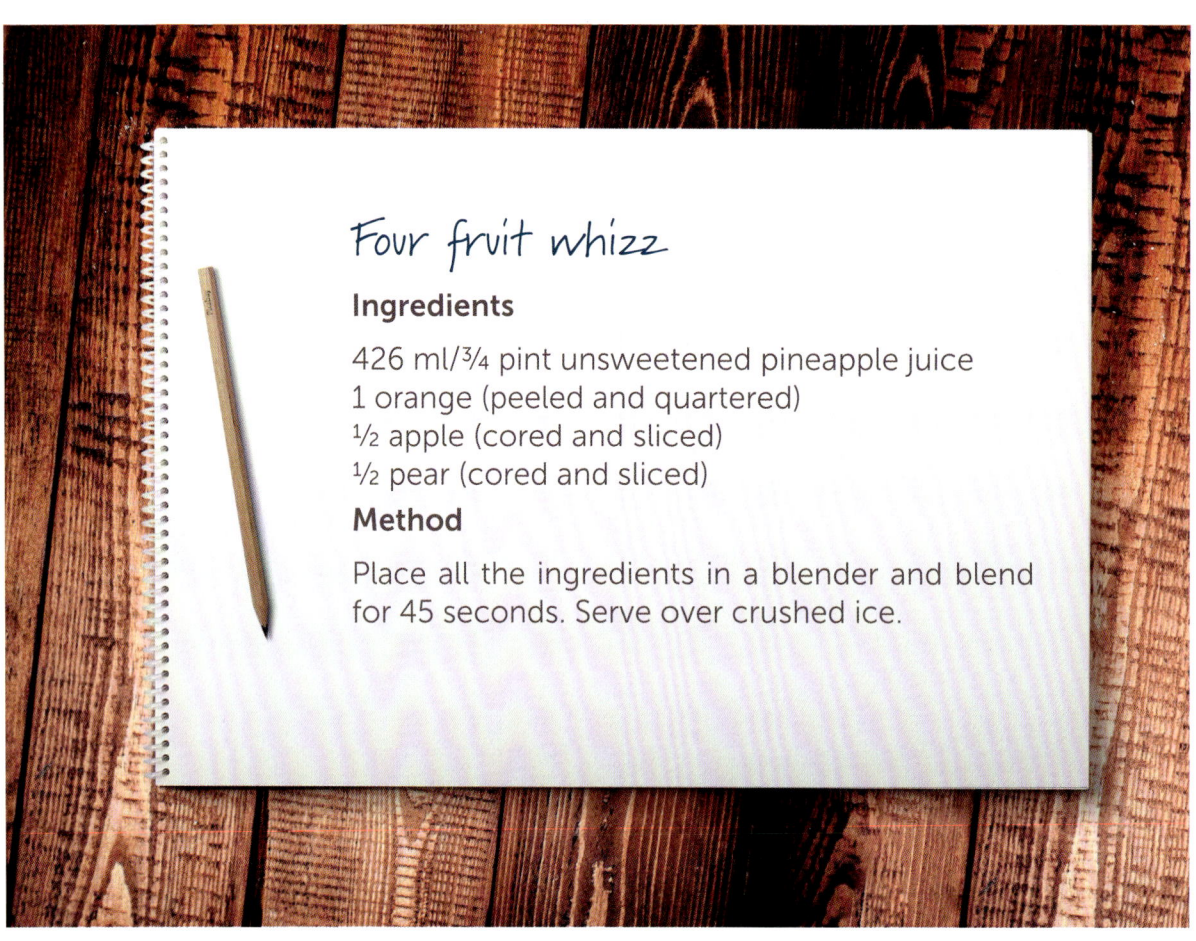

Four fruit whizz

Ingredients

426 ml/¾ pint unsweetened pineapple juice
1 orange (peeled and quartered)
½ apple (cored and sliced)
½ pear (cored and sliced)

Method

Place all the ingredients in a blender and blend for 45 seconds. Serve over crushed ice.

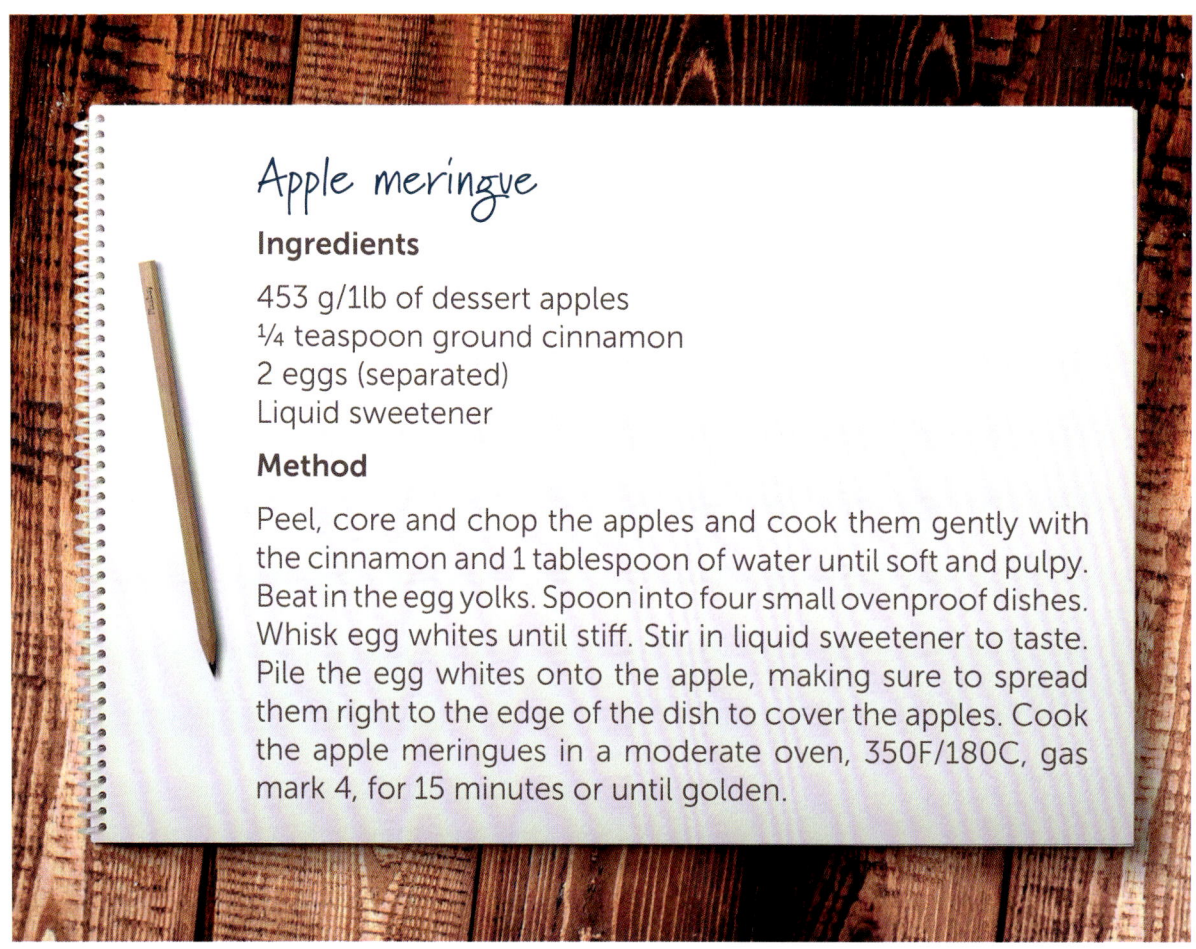

Apple meringue

Ingredients

453 g/1lb of dessert apples
¼ teaspoon ground cinnamon
2 eggs (separated)
Liquid sweetener

Method

Peel, core and chop the apples and cook them gently with the cinnamon and 1 tablespoon of water until soft and pulpy. Beat in the egg yolks. Spoon into four small ovenproof dishes. Whisk egg whites until stiff. Stir in liquid sweetener to taste. Pile the egg whites onto the apple, making sure to spread them right to the edge of the dish to cover the apples. Cook the apple meringues in a moderate oven, 350F/180C, gas mark 4, for 15 minutes or until golden.

Guide to Eating Out

Enjoying life!

Eating out is undeniably one of life's pleasures. It's usually a chance to take a break from the kitchen and enjoy a get together with friends and/or family to share conversation and good times.

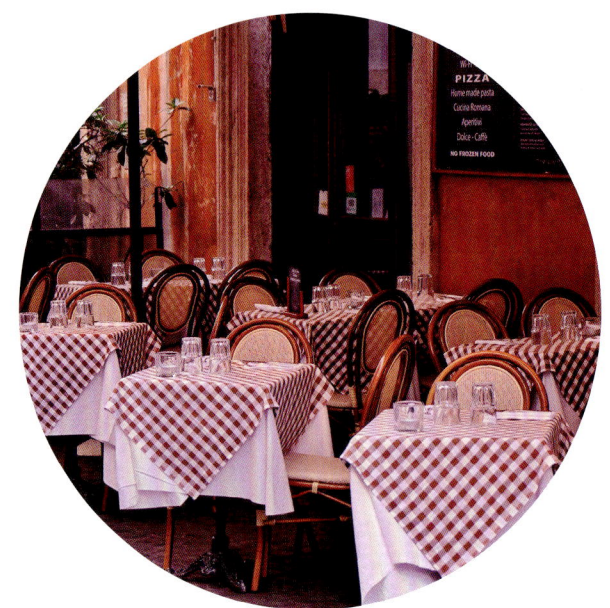

When you are on a diet... going out for a meal can be challenging. Let's face it, announcing that you're 'on a diet' is not the best feeling in the world; chances are you might even be a bit embarrassed. But the good news is you really don't have to say a word about dieting.

Whether it's English, Thai, Indian, Chinese, Turkish, Italian, Greek or any other type of restaurant; there will be dishes on the menu that you can eat. Follow my tips in this chapter and you will be able to keep on your healthy eating plan without anybody even realising.

Please remember, it's not the occasional meal that spoils your diet, it's when you start to over-indulge on daily treats that weight loss stops and weight gains begin.

In this chapter

Tips for eating out

What to drink

What to choose for starters and mains

What to choose for dessert

> **ALLERGY DISCLAIMER**
>
> Anyone with known or unknown, food intolerances or food allergies must take responsibility for food choices associated with this guidance.
>
> I will not assume any liability for adverse reactions from any of the foods listed in this book.

Tips for eating out

- Have a bowl of soup before you leave home and maybe a small amount of protein like chicken so you are not very hungry when you get to the restaurant. This is a good tip because you may not like all the choices on the menu and be tempted to make poor choices from a diet point of view. You may also have to wait a long time before the meal arrives

- Drink lots of water with your meal, you will feel full sooner and result in you eating much less food

- Choose very carefully from the menu

- Chew your food slowly – you will be satisfied with much less

- Talk a lot! It's surprising how much less you eat when you talk

- You can save up your alcohol allowance (one alcoholic drink a day) so you can choose from low carbohydrate lagers and red, white or rosé, wines

- Use low calorie mixers

- Dilute your wine with water or low calorie mixers for a longer drink

- If there's an opportunity to do some dancing, get on the dance floor and burn off some calories

- When you arrive home after the meal, always remember to eat a small amount of cucumber, which has been soaked in vinegar. Cucumber is a natural diuretic and the vinegar is an acid, which will help if you have eaten anything containing fat with the meal. (There could be extra fats, during the cooking process, that you are not aware of)

- If at the end of the meal you would like a coffee, please remember no sugar (sweeteners are permitted)

- If you're not keen on the main courses on offer you could ask for a double portion of your choice from the starter or vice-versa

- If you must have a pasta dish, choose one that comes in a tomato based sauce rather than a cream based sauce

What to drink

- Red, white or rosé, wine
- Any low carbohydrate lager or low calorie soft drink
- Low calorie lime or blackcurrant with water
- Decaffeinated tea or coffee
- Herbal tea
- Still water

Note: Please avoid spirits, liqueurs or cocktails — they can be very high in calories

What to choose for starters and mains

Choose	Avoid
Proteins like: eggs, steak, chicken, seafood, salmon (any other fish like tuna or sea bass for example), any other lean meats	Fried foods. Better to choose grilled, poached/boiled or roasted
Salads with ingredients from your allowed foods list. No dressing – except for a touch of olive oil (taken from your daily fat allowance) and balsamic vinegar	Potatoes
Vegetables (from the allowed list on page 99)	Rice/pasta
Clear soups	Sauces (if you can't live without the sauce get the waiter to serve it separately in a jug so you can control how much to add)
Garlic mushrooms	Mayonnaise (a tiny amount if used from your daily fat allowance)
Fresh fruit i.e. grapefruit or fruit salads	Dishes swimming in butter or oil
	Pasta with a creamy sauce*
	Bread (including garlic bread, bread sticks, pitta, naan, chapatis, dough balls)*
	Pancakes (for example with crispy duck) if you must, one pancake only*

*If you must have one of the flour based foods, such as bread and pasta; only have a small portion.

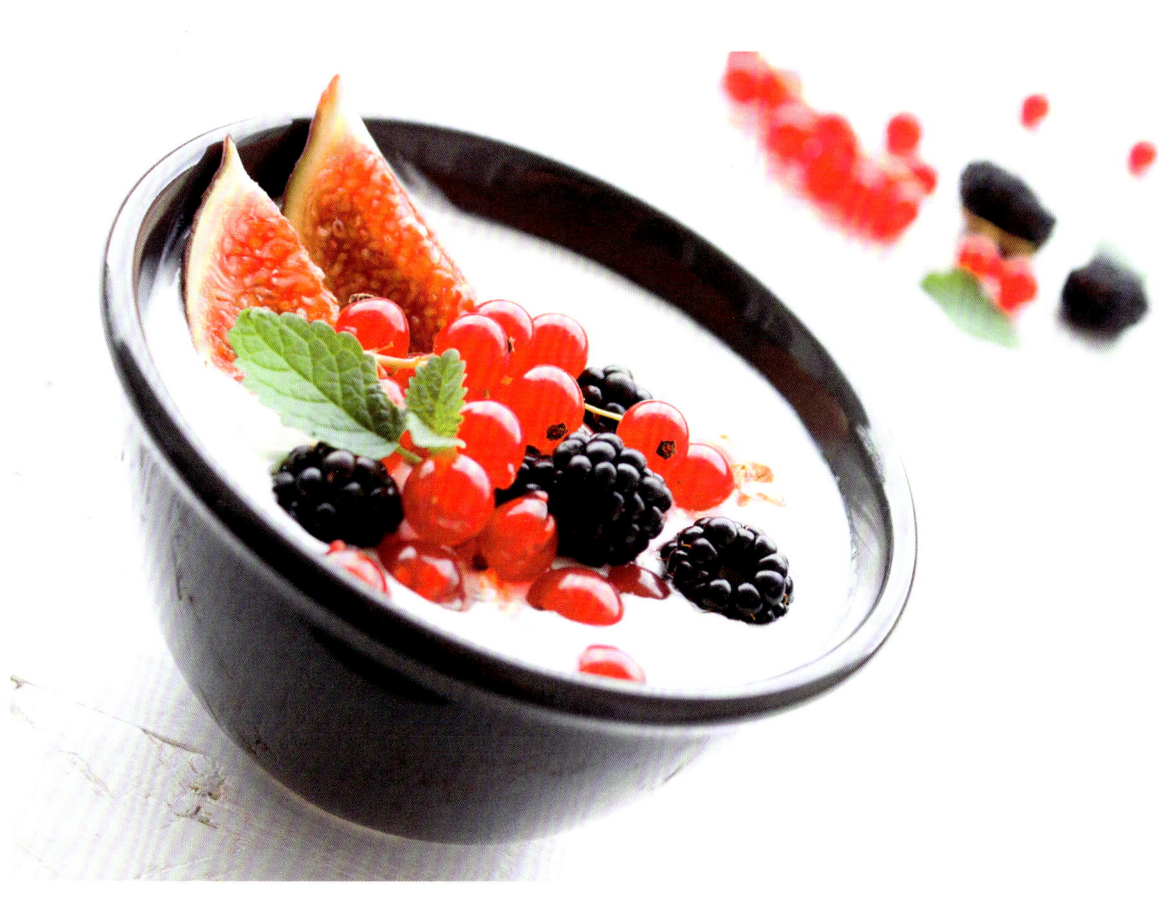

What to choose for dessert

Choose	Avoid
Fresh fruit salad	Ice cream
Strawberries and cream (tiny portion of cream)	Cream (a tiny portion is ok)
Melon	Cakes
Pineapple	Pastries
Natural organic yoghurt	Pancakes
	Sweet sauces
	Any form of sugar including honey and syrup

Acknowledgements

This is my third book and the one most dear to my heart because it has the power to transform the lives of the many millions of women suffering with PCOS.

Whilst it carries my name as author, the book is the result of a lot of collaboration with all sorts of people. It's the culmination of many hours of individual effort and focus for which I offer my heartfelt thanks to everyone involved.

Firstly, I'd like to thank Sasha McDonnell who did everything possible to help; both by contributing her own story to the book (see page 117) and by using her PCOS network in the PCOS community to help me find volunteers to trial endless diet and lifestyle interventions, over three long years! (See page 35). Sasha was my rock really, and without her help setting up the volunteer group, none of this would have happened.

And to Andy, Sasha's husband, for sharing his story too. His is a lone, but important voice in the book, telling the story of what it's like to be a loving husband or partner trying desperately to support their loved one who is often living a nightmare (see page 120).

And to the 100 volunteers from PCOS support groups who showed unstinting commitment, giving their time and focus to endless hours, days and months trialling countless diets and lifestyle 'tweaks'. There are too many to mention by name but without them there would be no Healthy Eating and Lifestyle Plan for PCOS for me to speak of and I am certain lots of little babies, some now nearly adults, would not have been born.

Since my Healthy Eating and Lifestyle Plan for PCOS was launched thousands of my PCOS sufferers have had great weight losses which has helped reduce their devastating symptoms and balance their hormones. Many of them were desperate for a baby, others just wanted to lead a 'healthy' life. I am delighted and thankful that some of these ladies have been generous enough to share their personal success stories to inspire others (see page 115).

Thanks also too, Derek Millard-Smith my legal adviser and K P Priest for his invaluable input and advice.

I'd also like to thank Alice de Matos for her writing contributions and for editing the book and managing the design and production. Thanks also to Carrie Leaver for her exceptional design talent and skill. Her use of colour and imagery has helped to translate the positivity and good news that this book brings to all PCOS sufferers – **there is an answer to PCOS.**

Last but not least, my son Damian, who kept reminding me of the need to get this book out there. The wind beneath my wings. Thank you.

Image credits

We have made every effort to credit photos where possible. With thanks to the following free stock image online libraries and contributors:

www.pixabay.com
https://www.pexels.com/u/public-domain-pictures/
Mali Maeder https://www.pexels.com/u/mali/
Kaboompics / Karolina https://www.pexels.com/u/kaboompics/
Lukas https://www.pexels.com/u/goumbik/
Kai Pilger https://www.pexels.com/u/kaip/
Tookapic https://www.pexels.com/u/tookapic/
Foodie Factor https://www.pexels.com/u/foodie-factor-162291/
Buenosia Carol https://www.pexels.com/u/buenosia-carol-116286/
Fancy Crave https://www.pexels.com/u/fancycrave-60738/
Breaking Pic https://www.pexels.com/u/breakingpic/
Hannah Nelson https://www.pexels.com/@hannah-nelson-390257
Beata Dudová https://www.pexels.com/u/beatadudova/
Skitter Photo https://www.pexels.com/u/skitterphoto/
Anthony https://www.pexels.com/u/inspiredimages/
Markus Spiske https://www.pexels.com/u/markusspiske/
www.flikr.com
Radoslaw Sikorski
Sergey Zolkin https://unsplash.com/@szolkin
Rawpixel.com https://unsplash.com/@rawpixel
Glenn Carstens-Peters https://unsplash.com/@glenncarstenspeters
Anna Simmonds https://unsplash.com/@annapress/collections
Anna Ogiienko https://unsplash.com/@panafotkas
Kate Krivanec https://unsplash.com/@katekrivanec
Joseph Gonzalez https://unsplash.com/@miracletwentyone
Tim Tiedemann https://unsplash.com/@timtied
Ylanite Koppens https://www.pexels.com
Illustrations and icons by Carrie Leaver

Notes

Experience shows that making notes of your daily eating habits and monitoring what you are doing encourages success.

Got a question? Feel free to send an email to **theanswertopcos@gmail.com** I am here to help.